Praise for *Tongue-Tied*

Having examined and treated newborns to adults with oral restrictions since the early 1980s, I have never seen such a complete and thorough study of the subject. Dr. Baxter has covered it all! His own personal experience was a great motivator to make this book a must-read for parents, physicians, dentists, lactation consultants, and therapists of all kinds.

Greg Notestine, DDS, AAACD
Founding Member and Past Director, International Affiliation of Tongue-Tie Professionals (IATP)

There can be no greater feeling than to see that I have been able to stimulate individuals like Dr. Baxter to add to the body of knowledge needed to educate the healthcare community as well as parents on the need to have tethered oral tissues evaluated for the many potential problems related to the tongue, which is not just a muscle, but a part of our body that can affect many of the body's systems, infant growth and development, speech and much more. Congratulations on writing this excellent book.

Larry Kotlow, DDS
Pioneer and World-Renowned Expert on
Tethered Oral Tissues

Tongue-Tied *is a revolutionary resource for parents, patients, and professionals alike. Such a detailed, comprehensive, and research-based resource has not existed until now! As a speech- language pathologist and certified orofacial myologist, this will be on the top shelf of my library and will be a resource I recommend to my colleagues, patients, and students. Thank you for filling this gap!*

Autumn R. Henning, MS, CCC-SLP, COM
Founder, TOTS Training

How refreshing to have a resource for parents and professionals based on clinical expertise and current research! Tongue-Tied is a straight-forward, no-nonsense approach to the influence of tethered oral tissues on both speech and feeding development.

Melanie Potock, MA, CCC-SLP
Author of Adventures in Veggieland *and co-author of* Raising a Healthy Happy Eater

As a surgical specialist and clinical researcher in the area of tethered oral tissues for close to 20 years, I have been waiting for a comprehensive text of this subject. Tongue-Tied is both a welcome addition and long overdue. It should serve as a concise guide for professionals as well as families seeking further knowledge on this topic. Thank you Dr. Baxter for moving our specialty forward!

Scott A. Siegel, MD, DDS, FACS, FICS, FAAP, DABLS
Oral and Maxillofacial Surgeon and Pioneer of Laser Lip- and Tongue-Tie Surgery

Dr. Baxter and his co-authors have done a remarkable job of tying together all of the current information on tethered oral tissues and their health impact in one place. This publication is the missing link and will help all of us who are involved in comprehensive patient care from newborns through underdiagnosed adults. Great job, Dr. Baxter and team!

Martin A. Kaplan DMD, DABLS
Pediatric Dentist and Director of Laser Dental Surgery for the American Board of Laser Surgery

TONGUE TIED

How a Tiny String Under the Tongue Impacts Nursing, Speech, Feeding, and More

RICHARD BAXTER, DMD, MS

with

Megan Musso, MA, CCC-SLP, **Lauren Hughes**, MS, CCC-SLP,
Lisa Lahey, RN, IBCLC, **Paula Fabbie**, RDH, BS, COM,
Marty Lovvorn, DC, and **Michelle Emanuel**, OTR/L, NBCR, CST
Foreword by **Rajeev Agarwal**, MD, FAAP

Tongue-Tied: How a Tiny String Under the Tongue Impacts Nursing, Speech, Feeding, and More

Published by Alabama Tongue-Tie Center
www.TongueTiedBook.com
Requests for information should be addressed to Alabama Tongue-Tie Center
Info@TongueTieAL.com
2480 Pelham Pkwy, Pelham, AL 35124

First Edition

Cover Design: Kostis Pavlou
Interior Design: Allan Ytac
Editors: Barbara Stark Baxter, Christine Ekeroth, Michael McConnell, and Taylor McFarland
Author photo by Christine Ekeroth

ISBN-13: 978-1-7325082-0-0
Printed in the United States of America

Publisher's Cataloging-in-Publication Data
Names: Baxter, Richard Turner, author. | Musso, Megan, author. | Hughes, Lauren, author. | Lahey, Lisa, author. | Fabbie, Paula, author. | Lovvorn, Marty, author. | Emanuel, Michelle, author. | Agarwal, Rajeev, foreword author.

Title: Tongue-tied : how a tiny string under the tongue impacts nursing , feeding , speech , and more / Richard Baxter, DMD, MS ; with Megan Musso, MA, CCC-SLP ; Lauren Hughes, MS, CCC-SLP ; Lisa Lahey, RN, IBCLC ; Paula Fabbie, RDH, BS, COM ; Marty Lovvorn, DC ; and Michelle Emanuel, OTR/L, NBCR, CST ; foreward by Rajeev Agarwal, MD, FAAP.

Description: Pelham, AL: Alabama Tongue-Tie Center, 2018.

Identifiers: ISBN 978-1-7325082-0-0 | LCCN 2018907841

Subjects: LCSH Tongue. | Pediatric otolaryngology. | Breastfeeding. | Speech. | Speech disorders in children. | Speech therapy for children. | Nutrition disorders in infants. | Nutrition disorders in children. | Pedodontics. | Children--Dental care. | BISAC MEDICAL / Pediatrics | MEDICAL / Dentistry / General | MEDICAL / Audiology & Speech Pathology | MEDICAL / Perinatology & Neonatology

Classification: LCC RF47.C4 .B39 2018 | DDC 618.92/09751--dc23

The author's royalties from this book will be donated to charity.

Disclaimer:

This publication is designed to provide general information about the subject matter covered and does not constitute clinical or medical advice. The author of this work has made every effort to use sources believed to be reliable to the standards generally accepted at the time of publication. This book is sold with the understanding that the author and publisher are not engaged in rendering professional services to the reader.

Knowledge and best practices in this field are constantly evolving. New research and experience broaden our understanding of the subject matter and may require changes in professional practices. Always consult with the current research and specific organizational policies and procedures prior to performing any medical or clinical procedures. The content is not guaranteed to be correct, complete or up-to-date.

Practitioners and researchers must always rely on their own experience and knowledge in evaluating and using any methods, charts, tables, procedures or other information described in this book. In using such information, they should be mindful of their own safety and the safety of others, including parties from whom they have a professional responsibility. If medical or any other expert assistance is required, the reader should seek the services of a professional. The information contained in this book is not intended to be a substitute for consulting with an experienced practitioner.

THE INFORMATION PROVIDED IS PROVIDED 'AS IS' AND NEITHER THE PUBLISHER, NOR THE AUTHOR,

For Hannah, Noelle, and Molly,
and for all of the patients we have had the privilege to treat.

Table of Contents

Acknowledgments

Richard Baxter, DMD, MS

First, I'd like to thank my wife, Tara, for her support of this project and her labor of love in raising our twin girls, both of whom had nursing difficulties with tongue- and lip-ties. Thank you to Dr. Taylor McFarland, Dr. Bobbie Baxter, Christine Ekeroth, Michael McConnell, and Lynn Richardson for spending countless hours editing and making suggestions to clarify our thoughts and make this project better in immeasurable ways. I'd like to thank the pioneers in the field of tongue-tie, who have made it easier for practitioners like me to care for these families. Thanks to Dr. Larry Kotlow, who has been so helpful answering questions, lecturing, and giving advice about treatment, both to me and thousands of other practitioners. Thanks to Dr. Marty Kaplan for his support, encouragement, and helpful courses on tongue-ties. Thanks to Dr. Bobby Ghaheri for writing his thought-provoking blog posts, reviewing the manuscript, and reaching out to dentists as an ENT to help educate and collaborate. Many of the thoughts and ideas presented in this book have been birthed out of interactions with and lectures given by these people, in addition to the knowledge gained from seeing patients struggling with tongue-ties every day in our office. Thank you to Megan, Lauren, Lisa, Paula, Marty, Michelle, and Rajeev who have contributed to this book and have devoted many, many hours to making this book a reality. I thank the Lord that He used our personal struggles with tongue-tie as a catalyst to help others with this condition.

Megan Musso, MA, CCC-SLP

I would like to express my gratitude to Dr. Baxter for allowing me to help with this book and for his patience and support as I juggled writing with life. To Courtney Gonsoulin, Diane Bahr, Melanie Potock, Autumn Henning, Kristie Gatto, and Dana Hearnsberger—thank you for providing me with a strong foundation in this area, encouraging me to be a voice for my patients, helping when the words wouldn't come, and being brave pioneers in our feeding world. To Kacie Peterson and Danielle Robinson—thank you for being part of the village and helping me be a better provider to our patients. I could not do my job without either of you. To my husband—thank you for believing in me and supporting me through all of my endeavors, and for never complaining when I bring work home. To the families that I have the honor of helping—thank you for fighting for your children and being their biggest advocates. Lastly, I owe all of my gifts and talents to God and am so thankful He chose me to fulfill His work through this extremely rewarding job.

Lauren Hughes, MS, CCC-SLP

First, I want to thank Dr. Baxter, not only for including me in this project, but also for all the help he's given me as I have gotten my practice off the ground. I wouldn't have my current experience or knowledge of tongue-ties if he hadn't included me in his process since our first meeting. Thanks to Autumn Henning for introducing me to tongue-ties from a speech-language pathologist's perspective, and for allowing me to use some of her valuable information in my chapters. Thank you to my friends and family for supporting me along the way as I step out in faith to establish my own private practice. Most importantly, I thank the Lord for using Dr. Baxter and each person who has contributed to this book to bring awareness to a topic that affects more families, children, and adults than any of us may know.

Lisa Lahey, RN, IBCLC

Thank you, Dr. Baxter, for your dedication to writing this book and asking me to contribute. It is my passion to share my experience, teach, and help parents and other professionals grow in their understanding and knowledge of breastfeeding and oral function at all ages. I would like to express my appreciation to the families, children, and adults I work with who teach me every day about complex feeding issues and perseverance. I wish to acknowledge the mentors who encouraged me to learn more about oral dysfunction and rehabilitation. I am particularly grateful for my loving husband and five children, who have supported me along the way and understand the sacrifice of my time and talents. I am grateful to God for blessing me with talents, skills, and a fulfilling vocation that enables me to help others find health and wellness.

Paula Fabbie, RDH, BS, COM

Thank you Dr. Baxter and all of the doctors and healthcare professionals for their trust and encouragement throughout the years. Their support enabled me to develop and grow my interest and abilities as an oral myologist/myofunctional therapist. I am grateful to my colleagues who share my high degree of altruism and have successfully co-treated many cases over the years. A very special thank you to Lorraine Frey RDH, LDH, BAS, COM, FAADH my co-author for her contributions, continued support, and excellent work in this essential emerging field. To my husband Joe, son Marc and his wife Laura for allowing me the time away from family for this passionate mission. Finally, to all the children and adults who have benefitted from this much needed therapy, thank you for allowing me to assist you on the road to wellness.

Marty Lovvorn, DC

I have great admiration for Dr. Baxter and his ability to positively impact future generations through his work. I am truly honored to be a part of his book. I sincerely appreciate Dr. Baxter's willingness to grow together in knowledge throughout this endeavor and am grateful for the opportunity to share a chiropractic perspective on the topic of tongue-tie conditions. I would like to thank my wonderfully supportive wife, Lindsey, for her unwavering spirit in sharing incredible passion for chiropractic and service to others. Her love for Christ, generous heart, and devotion to raising our two beautiful children inspires me daily. Most importantly, I would like to thank my Lord and Savior, Jesus Christ, for blessing all those involved in this book with the gifts to enhance the lives of others and help them achieve optimum health.

Michelle Emanuel, OTR/L, NBCR, CST

I am grateful for my 3 children, Eric Henry, Marin Elise and Ella Ann, as well as the thousands of babies I have evaluated and treated over the past 22 years or so. Both parenting and being a neonatal/pediatric occupational therapist have shaped and informed any expertise I have. I am grateful for my other teachers, Loren "Bear" Rex, Stephen Porges, Sue Ricks, many, many residents, fellows and attending neonatologists and neurologists during my hospital career and therapy colleagues who challenged my thinking and encouraged me to develop thoughts and contributions of my own. Thank you, Dr. Baxter, for putting this "team" together for the greatest benefit of the babies and families navigating their way through the TOTs world.

All of the proceeds from this book will be donated to charity for work locally and in the most impoverished areas around the world. We truly want this book to help educate parents and healthcare providers. Please share this book with your healthcare providers and other parents who might benefit from knowing more about this very common condition, and know that the profits are going to a worthy cause.

Foreword

Rajeev Agarwal, MD, FAAP

It is a great honor and privilege to be invited to write the foreword to this much-needed comprehensive and educational publication regarding issues surrounding the evaluation, diagnosis, and management of oral ties. I have been working in this field for more than 10 years and have often wished for a collective, comprehensive, and balanced document that I could share with my pediatric colleagues as well as patients and families, which outlines the past, present, and future issues associated with these very common diagnoses.

Pediatricians are charged with the responsibility of quickly and accurately identifying alterations to the most vital of biological functions in the newborn, including breathing, feeding, growth, and development. Feeding is a dynamic, multifaceted process encompassing physiology and anatomy, infant oral-motor function, and issues related to the primary caregiver, which is most often the breastfeeding mother. My interest in the effects of oral ties was ignited by the overwhelming volume of breastfeeding dyads failing to achieve reasonable feeding goals.

Over the past several decades, bottle-feeding has become the accepted answer for pediatricians when faced with slow weight gain and breastfeeding difficulties in infants. Although supplementation is often useful for meeting weight-gain goals and preventing post-birth complications and longer hospital stays, early identification of barriers to breastfeeding could surely increase the success rate for nursing dyads. Time is of the essence in the early postpartum period, and feeding difficulties should be thoroughly vetted to aid mothers in the successful institution of a breastfeeding relationship.

My interest in oral ties has taken root in this uncharted territory over the past 20 years of primary pediatric practice, and it is only in recent years that other professionals from a variety of specialties have begun to recognize oral restrictions as contributing to poor breastfeeding outcomes. Though my interest started with dysfunctional milk extraction in newborns, it has been easy to see how the oral ties affect an individual over his or her lifetime, along with compensatory mechanisms, which sometimes help the individual enough that the procedure is not warranted, but often do not help enough, which leads to a lifetime of functional deficits.

I often reflect back on my early medical training. I was taught very complicated algorithms for the diagnosis and management of rare diseases, but the seemingly simple issue of oral ties and feeding went unidentified or ignored. Sadly, the same is true for most pediatric residency programs even today, despite the overwhelming evidence demonstrating the benefits of breastfeeding to infant health and well-being.

Over the years, these diagnoses have also been burdened with a lot of myths, mysteries, and superlative claims that have divided pediatric care communities. Because so many specialties have "owned" the diagnosis and have put their spin on it, it has become like the proverbial blind men and the elephant! Everybody has something to say about it, but no one has yet presented the big picture effectively.

There has been mounting resistance, primarily grounded in misunderstanding, from pediatric care providers regarding evaluating, diagnosing, and managing oral ties, especially the more elusive posterior tongue-ties. The absence of standardized diagnostic criteria and management pathways, primarily related to the lack of published, quantifiable outcomes, have hampered the understanding of these conditions and given way to ambiguity and variation in management techniques. The concern among pediatric professionals is that "too many" infants are having frenectomy procedures and may not "need them." How do we identify need? How do we measure outcomes? How do we develop standardized procedures to create appropriate and safe inclusion criteria? Are tongue-ties a "new problem" or have they been an unrecognized, underdiagnosed problem? The sudden increase in the incidence of diagnosed tongue-ties, coupled with a steep incline in providers performing these procedures, has led to great controversy among those within the medical and breastfeeding communities.

Hopefully, this text will serve to examine, unify, and clarify information, creating a valuable and useful resource for parents and professionals alike. This book is comprehensive, organized, and well-written, but most importantly, it is balanced. It may be instrumental in increasing awareness, knowledge, and comfort regarding oral ties and associated issues for pediatric care providers, scope-of-practice concerns, and education in medical training programs. As I often state in many of my lectures, "Your eyes do not see what your mind does not know . . . but once you have seen it, it is impossible to unsee."

Introduction:
Why Write a Book About Tongue-Ties?

Imagine for a moment that you are born nearsighted (as all babies naturally are), but your nearsightedness (myopia) never self-corrects over time. Some readers may not have to stretch their imaginations much to do so, as this is their reality. When nearsighted as a young child, everything seems fine; toys, food, and loved ones are all nearby. However, behind the scenes, this limitation is slowly making everyday tasks more and more challenging. The child is largely unaware, as he assumes that what he is experiencing is shared by everyone and is therefore "normal," just as a person who is born colorblind will assume that the way he sees is normal. The nearsighted child will start to modify his actions to accommodate his unrecognized limitation, such as getting closer to the TV or sitting in the front of the room at school to be able to see the whiteboard more clearly. Although often diagnosed before age 12, sometimes it is not until that child is 16 years old and fails the vision portion of a driving test that he realizes he needs glasses! Thanks to a simple diagnosis via an eye examination and straightforward treatment with a pair of glasses, the world is now available in high definition. For the first time, that child can see leaves on trees! What wonders await!

An undiagnosed and uncorrected tongue-tie (also known as ankyloglossia) can follow a course similar to that of undiagnosed and uncorrected nearsightedness. More and more often, the effects of a tongue-tie are recognized early due to nursing, feeding, or speech difficulties, but sometimes the diagnosis still slips through the cracks and goes unidentified until adolescence or even adulthood.

Many adults reading this may experience sleep-disordered breathing, migraines, neck or shoulder pain, and difficulty with swallowing or speech. Any of these things coupled with a history of feeding and/ or speech problems as a child warrant an evaluation by a trained dental or medical professional for restricted tongue movement due to a persistent tongue-tie.

Although education related to the topic of tongue-ties is improving, the impact of such a restriction can still be excused or even ignored. With feeding difficulties, for instance, it might be said that the child is "easily distractible" or is "a picky eater." With breastfeeding difficulties, the mother might be told that "It is supposed to hurt for six weeks," or "You'll build calluses with time so it won't hurt so much," or "Your baby is just a lazy nurser." Such advice is often well-intentioned and meant to be encouraging, but it ignores the problem or fails to even recognize the problem at all. The real problem may well be a tongue-tie. Years of a person's life may be spent accommodating this unrecognized limitation when the actual process of diagnosing and treating a tongue-tie can be safe, simple, and straightforward, much like we saw for the nearsighted child above. Similar to the nearsighted child who isn't even aware of what he is missing, a life with an unrestricted tongue can open the door to a whole new world of speaking, eating, and many other invaluable human experiences.

The process of diagnosing a tongue-tie involves taking an in-depth history, completing in-person pretreatment assessments, and examining the oral cavity and head and neck structures. This process can be confusing for patients as well as providers. Our goal in writing this book is to make the process of diagnosing and treating tongue-ties safe, simple, and straightforward for practitioners as well as more easily accessible to patients, as the number of providers comfortable diagnosing and treating them increase.

On both a personal and professional level, my life has been deeply impacted by tongue-ties. I had a tongue-tie that went undiagnosed into adulthood, and my twin daughters both had tongue-ties. I've learned that such a thing shouldn't come as a surprise—predisposition to tongue-tie is a genetic trait, and it is common. When my tongue-tie was first recognized, I was training to become a dentist, and it was brought to my attention only as a possible cause of some minor gum recession. Even after my dental education at a great school, I did not know there were other problems the tongue-tie could cause, but I later learned that I had several.

Some researchers estimate the prevalence of tongue-tie to be between 4% and 10% of the population, but the actual number may be higher because most studies don't take into account posterior tongue-tie (discussed in detail later). It is likely that someone you know is affected by this condition and does not even know it. A tongue-tie can be the hidden reason behind nursing difficulties in babies, feeding problems in toddlers, speech issues in children, and even migraines or neck pain in adults. Is tongue-tie the cause of all the world's ills? No. But it is often overlooked, misdiagnosed, and written off by many healthcare providers. My hope is that this book and the stories within it will help encourage more healthcare providers, educators, parents, and patients to recognize that this condition is worth understanding and treating. Let's begin this journey together.

CHAPTER 1

∞

What Is a Tongue-Tie, Anyway?

I grew up with a tongue-tie and never knew I had one (and maybe you or someone close to you did, too). I finished dental school and pediatric dentistry residency without ever receiving a single lecture on tongue-tie. A tongue-tie must not be important or cause much trouble if it is not taught in dental schools, medical schools, or residency programs, right? Is it all just a myth? Is diagnosing and treating tongue-ties a fad or a way for surgeons to make money? This book is my humble attempt to help parents of children with tongue-ties, healthcare professionals, and even affected adults realize the implications of an untreated or poorly treated tongue-tie. If you're a provider and a skeptic, go ahead and skip to Chapter 9 for the research and evidence on tongue-ties and breastfeeding. Otherwise, continue reading with an open mind, and see the new paradigm that is emerging regarding tongue-ties.

The condition known as ankyloglossia has been around for thousands of years. There have been dozens of definitions proposed, and most contain similar elements, involving visual criteria, developmental origins, and functional limitations. Recently, the International Affiliation of Tongue-Tie Professionals (IATP, and yes, that is a real organization!) agreed on a succinct definition that encompasses the different presentations seen with tongue-tie. It states that tongue-tie is "an embryological remnant of tissue in the midline between the undersurface of the tongue and the floor of the mouth that restricts normal tongue movement."[1] This means it is a tight string of tissue under the tongue that can prevent the tongue from functioning properly. Most people have a frenum or string of some kind under the tongue, so many professionals consider a tongue-tie to be normal or a variant of normal. That's why the definition includes a caveat about "restricting normal tongue movement." There has to be a functional limitation in addition to an anatomical finding when you look under the tongue, in order for the oral structures to meet the criteria for a tongue-tie. If the tongue appears tied, it is important to assess what function has been impacted. Functional deficits may have been blamed on other factors ("He just gets distracted while nursing," or "He is a picky eater," when he is actually having difficulty with basic functional movement of the tongue), so asking specific questions is important. Often a patient can appear as if he is getting by just fine with his tongue restricted, or a baby can be gaining weight, so the parents are told "He's fine" (even with many other tongue-tie–related symptoms significantly affecting quality of life). We want babies, children, and adolescents not just to survive or be "fine," but to thrive and live without restrictions and compensations in nursing, feeding, speech, and more. No parent wants mediocrity for their baby or child. We want them to be the best they can be and live to their fullest potential. Something as simple as releasing a tongue-tie can be one part of helping a child reach his or her potential and achieve normal development.

> *There has to be a functional limitation in addition to an anatomical finding under the tongue in order to meet the criteria for a tongue-tie.*

Conversely, the tongue may not visually appear tied, but the baby, child, or adult may still exhibit symptoms of a tongue-tie. In this case, it is important to investigate further because it might be a variant known as a posterior tongue-tie. We have seen countless patients who have suffered from many of the symptoms of a tongue-tie and have been told by a healthcare provider that they do not have one; yet after the posterior tongue-tie is released, we often see the symptoms improve. Nursing improves, feeding improves, speech improves, and sleep improves, and often those results are immediate and not attributable to any other factor. Other tissues can also be restrictive or considered tied, leading to problems in the mouth. Examples of such tissues include a labial frenum (when restricted, it is known as a lip-tie), or even the cheek or buccal frena (when restricted, they are known as buccal-ties). These other ties are discussed along with traditional tongue-ties later in this book.

Now that we understand what a tongue-tie is, let's explore what a tongue-tie does. Imagine if your first pair of running shoes had the laces tied together. You try to run around the track, but you struggle. Could you eventually make it around? Yes, most likely. But would you fall to the ground, go slowly, or lose your balance at times? Almost certainly. Once someone points out that the laces are tied together and then unties or cuts the strings, now you can run faster and unhindered, and you didn't even realize that the laces weren't supposed to be tied together! This analogy illustrates the impact of living with a tongue-tie. Often many benefits of a tongue-tie release are realized after removal of the restriction, but a tongue-tie release alone will not provide the full benefits. Our fictitious runner who now has full mobility of her feet will be a bit awkward at first, running with two separate shoes and laces, but she will adapt quickly with coaching and time. Surgical treatment combined with speech, feeding, and myofunctional therapy for patients of all ages, as well as lactation support for babies, are goals that could lead to better outcomes. If you have walked around with your shoes tied together, your muscles and skills are not fully developed, and compensations need to be undone. The tongue is a muscle and, just as your legs would need to re-learn how to walk, the tongue muscle memory must be re-trained to do the proper movements and patterns to allow it to chew, talk, and swallow.

The tongue is a complex organ composed of eight muscles that are involved in feeding, breathing, speaking, sleep, posture, and many other essential functions. Ideal tongue function and muscle rest postures also provide a mold for proper growth and development of the dental arches and facial/airway development.

After completion of oral development in the fetus, a thin membrane called a frenum or frenulum underneath the tongue remains. This string of tissue varies in length, thickness, position, and elasticity. If the frenum is too short, too thick, too high up on the tongue, or too inelastic (or often a combination of these factors), the baby, child, or adult can have issues with feeding, speech, and more. Some ties are hidden underneath the outer mucosal layer and are not readily visible. The mouth is also naturally a part of the body considered more mysterious than others because its contents are hidden. When the body has an external congenital issue, such as fused fingers, it is typically easier to diagnose and receive treatment for that than for a congenital disability of the oral structures. Some anatomical defects of the mouth are well understood, their assessment is routine and treatment for them is widely accepted. For example, most providers recognize a cleft palate and understand that it can cause issues with nursing, feeding, and speech. When it comes to an anatomical defect with the tongue, however, many do not understand how to diagnose such a defect, nor do they associate the functional issues with the anatomical defect.

Embryology

A tongue-tie results from a failure of the tissue under the tongue to completely resorb during development, which is a process known as apoptosis (programmed cell death) around the 12th week in utero.[2,3] The frenum results when the tongue moves posteriorly (backward) from the primitive jawbone, and it holds the tongue in the correct position. It is then supposed to disappear.[2] A common example of apoptosis is the gradual disappearance of the tadpole-like tail that occurs as the human embryo develops. A fault in the apoptotic process can leave a string under the tongue that is connected too high on the gum and under the surface of the tongue. Another variation of faulty apoptosis occurs when the string has mostly disappeared, but the tissue is tighter or less elastic than it should be. This more restrictive tissue can lead to problems similar to those of the classic tongue-tie. The example above of webbed fingers, also known as syndactyly, also results from a failure of tissue apoptosis.

A Brief History of Tongue-Ties

The condition of tongue-tie and the process of releasing the tongue was noted in early Japanese writings, other historical documents, and even the Bible. Moses was thought to be tongue-tied, as it reads in Exodus 4:10 that he was "slow of speech and of tongue" (ESV). Mark 7:35 tells of a deaf man Jesus healed who also had a speech impediment. It says that "his ears were opened, his tongue was released, and he spoke plainly" (ESV). Some translations even mention "the string of his tongue" (KJV).

For a long period, the tongue-tie was released without a second thought and was seen for what it is—a restrictive piece of tissue that holds the tongue down and keeps it from doing its important work. In the 1600s, frenotomy was widely known. An obstetric textbook from 1609 states: "One should also gently pass the finger under the tongue to find if they have the band...the surgeon consulted to this business will remove it with a scissors tip without risk."[4] Louis XIII, the King of France born in 1610, had the procedure done. "Seeing that he had trouble nursing we looked into his mouth. It was seen that the tongue-string was the cause. At five in the evening it was cut in three places by M. Guillemeau, the king's surgeon."[4] Around this time and prior, midwives would keep one fingernail sharp so that if a newborn baby had a tongue-tie, they could release the tongue without the use of instruments (which they were not allowed to use).[5] There are wood carvings from 1620 that reveal Fabricius' technique for releasing the tongue, with a baby swaddled and the tongue held with a handkerchief. In 1666, a "tongue lifter" was invented by Scultetus and improved upon in 1680 by Mauriceau. In 1774 (just before the American Revolution), Petit improved upon these designs and invented the grooved director that is still used today.[4]

Releasing the tongue appears to be one of the oldest surgical procedures still being performed today, although it used to be far more common than it is at present. Nursing issues and speech issues including stuttering, speech delay, and lisping were also seen as tongue-tie problems and were treated by cutting the string without hesitation.[5]

From 1830 to 1841 a great wave of surgeries swept through France, Germany, and England,[5] leading many people to seek out surgeons for all kinds of issues. Some surgeries were truly helpful, while others were less so. Once people realized in the 1850s that surgery wasn't the best option in all cases, they began to think it wasn't helpful in any case. The metaphorical "throwing the baby out with the bathwater" occurred, and, unfortunately, surgically releasing the tongue fell out of favor—not due to a lack of evidence, but by cultural choice.

> *Releasing the tongue appears to be one of the oldest surgical procedures still being performed today.*

In the past, if a mother was unable to nurse her baby, the family would employ a wet nurse to nurse the baby, or the baby would die due to lack of nourishment. Historically, in some eras breastfeeding was regarded as something the "common people" did, so royalty or the elite would hire wet nurses instead of breastfeeding. The practice of wet nursing declined in the 1800s, but many still employed them to feed their babies. As infant formula was developed and became safer in the early 1900s, marketing campaigns by companies such as Nestlé® began promoting their formula products and implying they were better than breast milk. These companies provided formula to hospitals so they could start the babies off on the right foot. Drinking from a bottle allowed the milk to fall into the baby's mouth with little effort, so nursing problems were treated with a bottle and formula. As formula feeding became more common, the tongue-tie wasn't treated at birth, and it would persist into toddler years, childhood, and adulthood. With tongue-ties resulting from dominant genes in many cases, successive generations had more and more tongue-tied people.

In recent decades there has been a resurgence in breastfeeding, along with a growing body of research supporting its benefits.[6–8] These include reductions in otitis media, asthma, eczema, obesity, diabetes, childhood leukemia, and SIDS.[6] We are also seeing more mothers initiating and having difficulty nursing their infants. A bottle won't tell you whether it has pain or a poor latch, but a mother is acutely aware of it every time the baby nurses. Many mothers experience painful nursing, with bleeding and cracked nipples, while their babies may experience poor weight gain, excessive gas, reflux, and a shallow latch. The response of many providers to such problems is still simply to offer the child a bottle with formula, and maybe some reflux medication. Some providers might fail to recognize these issues or even dismiss them outright, forcing patients to look for answers elsewhere.

A bottle won't tell you whether it has pain or a poor latch, but a mother is acutely aware of it every time the baby nurses.

In recent years, there has been a steady rise in the number of people asking for help in online forums or social media platforms. Mothers with difficulties related to breastfeeding have formed large online communities where they share tips and information. As a result, there has been a renewed interest in the diagnosis and treatment of tongue-tie. Treating tongue-tie is a surgical procedure that can offer enormous benefits with very little risk to patients in need. I encourage practitioners, however skeptical, to read on, because patients are out there seeking answers for their struggles, and tongue-tie may well be a contributing factor that you could learn to recognize and treat or refer for treatment.

CHAPTER 2

---∞---

It's Complicated—
The Misunderstood Tongue-Tie

To date, more than 500 articles on tongue-ties have been published in peer-reviewed journals, according to a PubMed search. Research on tongue-ties has historically stirred up disagreements about the definition, assessment, and diagnosis of a tongue-tie, the means of measuring the effects of releasing the tie, and the complexities related to the ethics of working on vulnerable babies. There are strong opinions on both sides of the debate as to the merits of releasing a tie. As mentioned previously, tongue-tie is similar to syndactyly, also known as webbed fingers. Syndactyly is a congenital deformity of fused tissues that may cause a limitation that can have a negative functional impact throughout life. As with the common practice of separating webbed fingers in the case of syndactyly, I do not believe the issue of tongue-tie release should be controversial. The primary difference between the two conditions is that the tongue-tie is relatively hidden and not easily assessed by an untrained provider. Once teeth erupt, to elevate the tongue and examine a baby properly may put you at risk for losing a finger, or at least being bitten! Additionally, the contemporary medical community has not studied the diagnosis or treatment of tongue-ties while in training.

Lactation consultants, who are often the first care providers to pick up on this issue, are not allowed to officially diagnose the presence of a tie per their practice guidelines. Speech therapists don't routinely check in the mouth and must receive special permission to perform an oral examination in school-based speech programs. Lactation consultants, speech therapists, and other health professionals also vary in their knowledge and familiarity of tongue-ties. Many training programs leave out or dismiss the idea that tongue-ties cause issues. The dentist is the physician of the mouth and should diagnose a restricted tongue during a soft tissue examination, but without proper education and training, ties often go undiagnosed by dentists as well.

As a board-certified and actively practicing pediatric dentist, I routinely see new patients who are 7 to 15 years old for whom I am the first person to mention to the parent that the child has a significant and functionally restrictive tongue-tie. Parents often wonder why no one ever told them their child was tongue-tied. After hearing this many times, I began to feel a responsibility to at least attempt to play a part in reducing the number of undiagnosed tongue-ties that are causing functional problems in children. I believe that it is not an indication of a lack of caring or poor training; rather, it is simply a gap in medical and dental education. Physicians learn much less about pathological conditions in the mouth than dentists, and dental training often focuses intensely on the teeth and gums. In dental school, students study oral pathology for countless hours and are tested on very rare conditions that may affect one in a million people, while something that may affect 1 in 10 is left out. My hope is that this book will help providers, parents, educators, and patients see that this seemingly minor condition can cause significant problems. Once the medical community as a whole recognizes this condition and understands how to diagnose and treat it, countless lives will be changed for the better. It is quite likely that every provider, once

Once the medical community as a whole recognizes this condition and understands how to diagnose and treat it, countless lives will be changed for the better.

educated about this common congenital abnormality will have the opportunity to identify a tongue-tie that is causing a functional limitation the very next day in practice!

Many professionals have strong and varied opinions regarding tongue-ties.[9] Some pediatricians believe that no tongue-ties affect breastfeeding, whereas some say that only classic ties (at or near the tip) affect breastfeeding. Others have seen the benefits of releasing anterior and posterior (or submucosal) tongue-ties. Lactation consultants have varying levels of training regarding tongue-ties, with some falling on different sides of the "release or do not release" debate. Some believe that classic anterior tongue-ties should be released when they are causing functional problems, but that posterior ties don't exist. Some breastfeeding specialists think that tongue-ties and nursing difficulties can be overcome with better positioning during nursing, and tongue-tie releases are rarely, if ever indicated.

However, many parents whose babies I have treated for posterior tongue-tie (after exhausting all other options) report marked improvement in nursing immediately after their child's tongue-tie release. One baby with a posterior tongue-tie and a restrictive lip-tie was consuming only 2 oz of breastmilk in 45 minutes during a weighted feed (weigh the baby, let them nurse, weigh again, and the difference is the amount of milk taken). Immediately after the procedure—and that was the only difference—he took 4 oz in 10 minutes of nursing (see photo of the posterior tongue-tie and laser release). That's an improvement from 1.3 mL/min to 12 mL/min after the procedure. A weighted feed is an objective measure, but it is also worth noting that subjectively the mother also experienced significantly less pain while nursing. This example is representative of patients in whom tongue tie releases are done correctly. Objective measures such as milk intake before and after nursing and hearing no clicking noises, coupled with subjective measures such as the mom noticing a deeper latch and less pain, confirm the fact that a posterior or submucosal tie did exist and was causing problems. This scenario repeats itself regularly in many

11

offices when releases are performed on babies who have posterior tongue-ties, and other practitioners report seeing the same results.

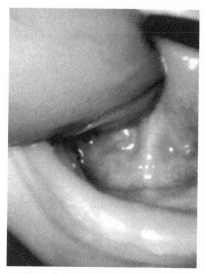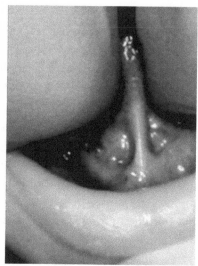

Aforementioned baby with posterior tongue-tie: elevation and two finger evaluation revealing the thick, restrictive tie.

We owe it to our patients to use the most up-to-date knowledge and best clinical judgment to help mother-infant dyads who are struggling with painful and inefficient nursing. There are multiple studies and blinded randomized controlled trials showing that releasing the tongue can help with breastfeeding issues.[10–20] In fact, no evidence-based research exists to show the non-effect from treatment of tongue-ties in infants struggling to nurse effectively. The only procedural harm that has been reported by these studies is minor bleeding, although more excessive bleeding is a possibility when scissors are used, or the cut is too deep, which highlights the need for proper training. The majority of studies support Buryk's assertion in the journal *Pediatrics* that the procedure is "rapid, simple, and without complications."[10] Interestingly, Dr. Kotlow, a pediatric dental practitioner, references a parody article about parachute safety,[21] and likes to ask in his lectures, "Who would like to participate in a randomized controlled trial to determine if a parachute works?" The response is of course silence. For some things that seem to clearly work, we don't need to subject others to harm so we can have a tidy research study. This is why there is such difficulty obtaining approval from ethics boards to perform randomized trials on infants; the potential benefit of tongue-tie release makes it unethical to deny that treatment to others for the sake of a study control group. Blinded randomized controlled trials and case studies have been conducted, however, and it is my hope that this book will convince the skeptics that diagnosis and treatment of tongue-ties can be of huge benefit to their patients.

The effects of a tongue-tie may last a lifetime. Some who have previewed this book have said it brought up traumatic memories of being teased in childhood, and they found it painful to read. If this is you, please know that it's never too late to have a tongue-tie released, and reading this book may help you to understand your situation better. The resources at the end may help you to find the right provider or support group for your situation.

This book provides an overview of the current thinking and research about tongue-ties and lip-ties as they affect patients throughout their lives. After you read this book, our hope is that the importance of correcting tongue-ties will be very clear to you, and you will find that your ability to help patients, parents, and perhaps even your family members is newly enhanced. In the Foreword, Dr. Agarwal wisely reminds us that the "eyes do not see what [the] mind does not know." Once you have the latest knowledge about tongue-ties in your mind, you will very likely be able to analyze your patients' related issues in a new context. So enjoy the journey of discovery presented here. Mothers and children are waiting for answers from their healthcare providers regarding health issues related to difficulties with nursing, eating, speaking, and many other areas of life that turn out to be affected by these abnormal structures.

Section 1: Nursing

T he following vignette is a composite of many of my patients' roller coaster experiences of emotions and doctor visits, and it is a story that is repeated in our office more often than we would like.

Baby Maggie was born full term at 40 weeks weighing 8 lb 2 oz to a first-time mom who had made the decision to breastfeed. In the hospital, when Maggie tried to latch, everything appeared to be normal. The lactation consultant came around and mom reported to her that nursing was pinching a little bit. The specialist reassured her that Maggie was just getting used to breastfeeding and that the positioning looked good. At home, however, Maggie was spitting up and burping all the time. She seemed more fussy than average, and she looked uncomfortable. At Maggie's first visit to the pediatrician, her mom was assured that some babies are just fussier than others.

But every feed was still a struggle, and Maggie was still spitting up a lot. The pain got worse, and at three weeks, Maggie still hadn't regained her birth weight. Her mom sought out a lactation consultant, who noted the latch looked good from the outside and that she seemed to be transferring milk well, so she gave her a nipple shield to help ease her discomfort.

Still frustrated and searching for answers, Maggie's mom posted her dilemma on Facebook, and a friend suggested she join a support group on Facebook and check out an online list of professionals who work with tongue-tied babies. As a last resort before switching to formula, mom decided to make the four-hour drive to the closest provider on the list. At the provider's office, he asked questions about the baby's and mom's symptoms, examined the baby's entire mouth using appropriate positioning and a headlight with magnification, and took pictures, pointing out the areas where tissues were restricted. Mom had all of her questions answered in detail.

After discussing the procedure, risks, benefits, aftercare exercises, and need for follow-up with a team of professionals, the provider used an ultra-precise laser to remove the restricted tissue under the lip and the tongue with minimal to no bleeding and no sutures. No general anesthesia or sedation was needed. A small amount of numbing jelly was used to help ease the discomfort. Immediately after the procedure, Maggie was taken to her mother in a private nursing room where she was able to nurse in seclusion. Mom noticed a deeper latch and less pain immediately, although Maggie seemed like she was not quite sure what to do with the new freedom in her tongue. After nursing, she did seem happier and more full. She had stopped making clicking noises, and she was finally feeding in a more relaxed position rather than being frustrated at the breast.

The next week, Mom had several visits with her lactation consultant, who helped with positioning, latch, and emotional support. Seven days after the procedure, Mom reweighed Maggie, who had gained a full pound! There were still some difficult feeds mixed with the good ones, but overall mom noticed that the improvement was holding. The hardest part was keeping up with the aftercare exercises four to six times a day to help the area heal properly. Even though the exercises were quick and as playful as possible, Maggie didn't like having mom's fingers in her mouth. Mom had more confidence that she could breastfeed Maggie, and the pain and stress they were both experiencing was much relieved. Maggie regained her weight and was back up to the 75th percentile by the third month.

This section is likely the most critical for many reasons. We'll start with how symptoms of a tongue-tie affect the mother and then the baby. Next, we will discuss the lip-tie and other oral ties. The role of the lactation consultant, assessment, compassionate care, the tongue-tie release, and what to do afterward will also be discussed. Finally, we'll conclude this section with a review of the published evidence. If the tongue-tie release occurs during the infant stage, a host of potential issues in the future can be prevented.

CHAPTER 3

---❦---

Tongue-Ties and Babies

The nursing relationship between mother and baby is vital, and the difficulties they experience can affect their bond and the baby's health during a critical time of development. Many mothers of tongue-tied babies experience excruciating pain from a poor latch. We have mothers in our office nearly every day who report severe pain when nursing. Moms know the benefits of breastfeeding, and they want to do it, but it may be so painful that they can't endure it long-term. Meanwhile, many well-meaning people in their circle advise them to give up, supplement, or pump exclusively if there are problems. Mothers try to push through the pain and reach out to professionals for help. Often if there is significant pain, there is a problem, and the most likely reason is that the baby is biting down on the nipple or using excessive vacuum pressure to try to extract milk. The most likely reason this happens is that the tongue isn't moving properly.

Babies have a reflex to bite if there is some object (nipple, bottle, finger, pacifier) between their gums and the tongue is not sticking out over the lower gum pad. If the tongue is restricted and unable to move forward to cup the nipple, covering the gum pad, the baby will bite down reflexively. That hurts. Pain, however, does not always indicate a tongue-tie, and many babies with a tongue-tie surprisingly do not cause pain during nursing for mom, but instead have other signs, such as a poor latch, poor seal, losing milk out of the corner of the mouth, and gagging while feeding. A tongue-tie release provider assesses all of these symptoms and tries to make the best decision for the infant and mother and only intervene when other options have failed. For this reason, if you are having nursing difficulty, it is important to first be evaluated by a knowledgeable International Board Certified Lactation Consultant (IBCLC). After breastfeeding has been assessed, and lactation interventions fail to address the issue, or a tie has been identified, an examination by a provider who is knowledgeable about tongue-ties should be considered.

> *If the tongue is restricted and does not cover the gum pad, the baby will bite down reflexively.*

Mother's Symptoms
>> Painful nursing
>> Poor latch
>> Cracked, creased, flattened nipples
>> Bleeding nipples
>> Lipstick shaped nipples
>> Poor breast drainage
>> Plugged ducts, engorgement, mastitis
>> Nipple thrush
>> Using a nipple shield
>> Feeling like feeding the baby is a full-time job

The consultation visit should include a review of the medical and feeding history and all the symptoms of the mother and the baby to get a full picture of where the issues lie. These symptoms are integral to determining whether or not to proceed with a tongue-tie release. Without this information, it is challenging to make an educated decision as to whether to treat or not. Other issues for mothers include bleeding, cracked, creased, or lipstick-shaped nipples. These are a result of a shallow latch, excessive biting, and pressure from the baby trying to get milk as best he or she can by using excessive force. If the baby has to use the lips and cheek muscles to create a vacuum, like sucking on a straw, this will extract milk inefficiently and also cause significant nipple damage. This damage can lead to wounded nipples, mastitis, or thrush. The ineffective latch can also lead to plugged ducts and poor breast drainage when milk is left over after feeding and breasts remain full.

A tongue-tied baby often will not receive enough milk to feel full, causing the baby to want to feed every 30 to 60 minutes. Babies with a tongue restriction will inefficiently suck and transfer milk and may feed for an hour at a time. To prevent engorgement or mastitis, a mother may have to use a breast pump to relieve the pressure of the excess milk the baby was unable to transfer and use her own milk in a bottle to top off and satisfy her baby. The triple feeding—feeding at breast, pumping, and feeding pumped milk by bottle or supplemental nursing system (SNS) at breast—often leaves the mother exhausted and frustrated with the process, and can lead to premature weaning of breastfeeding. Most often, moms report to us that it "feels like a full-time job just to feed him!"

Babies are highly adaptable and try to get milk any way they can. There is no such thing as a baby who "does not want to eat" or a baby who is "just not interested." They certainly may be tired from exerting so much effort to nurse, but saying they desire not to take milk or not feed is not the case. It is the baby's biological need to breastfeed for both nutrition and nurturing. Phrases such as "That's just how some babies are," or "Some mothers [or babies] just can't breastfeed" should be a red flag to families that the practitioner may not be up-to-date on current breastfeeding or tongue-tie information and should lead the parent to search for other answers. Just because something is common does not mean it is healthy or normal.

> *Moms report to us that it "feels like a full-time job just to feed him!"*

21

Tongue-Tied Baby's Issues

- » Poor latch at breast or bottle
- » Falls asleep while feeding
- » Slides on and off the nipple when feeding
- » Cries often/fussy often
- » Reflux symptoms
- » Spits up often
- » Clicking or smacking noises when eating
- » Gagging or choking when eating
- » Gassy burps and toots
- » Poor weight gain
- » Biting/chewing the nipple
- » Pacifier falls out easily or won't stay in
- » Milk dribbles out of the mouth when eating
- » Short sleeping
- » Mouth breathing, snoring, noisy breathing
- » Congested nose
- » Milk coming out of the nose
- » Frustration at breast or with bottle
- » More than 20 minutes per feeding required after newborn period
- » Eating more frequently than every 2 to 3 hours

As previously mentioned, babies can experience poor weight gain because they are consuming less milk per suck than would a non-tongue-tied baby. They are using muscles other than the tongue, such as cheek or lip muscles, to get milk, and they become more tired and burn more calories trying to eat than does a baby free of restrictions. Many (but not all) babies we see have trouble regaining birth weight or staying on the growth curve. Ideally, babies should gain their birth weight back within 10 days, although some still take longer. But we have some babies at our office

Just because something is common does not mean it is healthy or normal.

who are one or even two months old and are not much heavier than their original birth weight.

We want to encourage parents to discuss feeding and weight issues with their pediatrician and seek help from a skilled IBCLC. Parents can weigh the baby if they suspect there may be an issue with weight gain. Lactation consultants will often assess a pre- and post-breastfeeding weight on a highly accurate digital scale to determine exactly how many milliliters of milk the baby takes from each breast during a feeding. Far too often, babies who are having trouble gaining weight are given formula or told to switch to bottle-feeding without investigating all of the potential causes of the issue. An IBCLC can best assess the mother's milk supply and feeding issues and design a feeding care plan to problem solve root causes and increase the mother's milk supply.

Often parents have commented that the child's doctor was unsure about how to assist with the breastfeeding issues, so formula was seen as a quick fix. A recent survey of pediatricians revealed that they have limited clinical lactation knowledge and training with breastfeeding management. The survey revealed pediatricians often receive as little as 3 hours of breastfeeding education per year during residency.[22] More education and training is key. A lack of education coupled with increasing patient loads and decreasing insurance reimbursements to primary care providers have only magnified this problem, as they reduce the amount of time the provider can spend with each patient to dig deep and ask probing questions.

Usually, if problems persist, the pediatrician will recommend pumping and bottle-feeding or simply formula and bottle-feeding. Some babies with a tongue-tie may see improvement with bottle-feeding, but many still have problems such as gassiness, fussiness, reflux, and spitting up. Many have milk dribble out the corner of the mouth when feeding, which results in having to wear a bib during feeding and developing a rash on the neck. Some babies on formula or expressed breast milk—if the mother is triple feeding (nursing, pumping, and feeding the expressed milk)—still have trouble gaining weight and are hospitalized. When this happens, they undergo all manner of invasive tests and procedures including swallow studies, GI scopes, ultrasounds, X-rays, and feeding tubes, which cost thousands of dollars and hours of stress and worry for the parents. Too often, babies in these intensive feeding programs are either not adequately assessed or never checked for a tongue-tie. Even if examined, many of those assessing for ties are not aware of the spectrum of presentations. The doctors also often fail to look beyond the baby and question mothers about the symptoms discussed above using a checklist or a questionnaire (see Appendix).

Ideally, this assessment would occur at the pediatrician's office during a routine check-up, with referral to a skilled lactation consultant for one-on-one therapy if there are issues.

Many of those assessing for ties are not aware of the spectrum of presentations.

Other symptoms exhibited in babies with tethered tissues are related to the poor latch. The lip-tie, or restrictive maxillary frenum, can very much affect nursing and a quality latch. If the baby has an ineffective seal on the breast (or bottle), there will be a clicking or smacking noise heard when the baby eats. This sound is a sign that air is entering the baby's mouth and the baby is swallowing pockets of air. These babies are literally eating air, a condition known as aerophagia.[23] If this happens during feeding, the baby will have a distended or hard belly, and be very gassy and fussy. The air either comes back up from the belly as big burps or spit-up, or passes through and is released as toots. The spit-up ranges from simple teaspoon-sized wet burps to large "I think he may have spit up everything he ate" vomits. Spit-up also creates massive amounts of laundry due to the need to repeatedly wash bibs, burp cloths, the baby's clothes, and mother's or father's clothes. This seemingly insignificant problem increases the burden of a tongue-tie on families. Many parents mention to us that their baby "toots like a grown man." The babies have excessive gas in their intestines and pass gas frequently. These babies are labeled as "colicky" or "fussy" and treated with gripe water or simethicone gas drops in an attempt to alleviate the excess gas instead of finding the cause of the gassiness. Certainly, there can be other causes of colic or reflux, but any baby displaying signs of either should be evaluated for a tongue- or lip-tie.

Dr. Scott Siegel, MD, DDS, FAAP (Fellow of the American Academy of Pediatrics), has been treating babies with tongue- and lip-ties in New York for almost 20 years and recently published a paper about aerophagia-induced reflux (AIR).[23] He describes a condition we just discussed, in which a baby with tongue-tie swallows or eats air and subsequently has reflux-like symptoms. In the study, Dr. Siegel treated 1,000 infants with reflux by merely releasing the tongue- and/or lip-tie, and 52.6% improved in their reflux symptoms so significantly that they were able to wean off or decrease their medications (such as Zantac® or Nexium®). Improvements were often seen within a week or two. Another 19.1% improved in their reflux symptoms but still needed medications. The last group, 28.3%, did not have any change in their reflux symptoms—pointing to another cause of their reflux. This study demonstrates the effectiveness of treating the restricted tongue in many cases of reflux. The concept of AIR should be put into practice for every baby who has signs and symptoms of reflux before medication is considered. Babies with reflux, choking, or spitting up should be checked for an anterior (classic) tongue-tie or a posterior submucosal tongue-tie that is restricting function and potentially causing the issue.

The Elusive Posterior Tongue-Tie

Some babies have difficulty nursing or bottle-feeding and have symptoms similar to those listed above, but when a parent or provider looks in the mouth, it appears normal at first glance. It is often by looks alone that many providers then diagnose the child as not having a tongue-tie. The mother is left confused, as she is still having issues related to nursing, which may or may not prompt her to look elsewhere for advice. The solution to catching these elusive posterior ties is simple—an oral examination including feeling underneath the tongue.

Some practitioners believe there is no such thing as a posterior tongue-tie. They say that it doesn't exist, or it doesn't cause problems. The name "posterior tongue-tie" does not accurately describe the finding (it is not in the back of the throat), but it is the most common terminology, so it will be used throughout this book. Of note, many babies may appear to have posterior ties, but if there are no symptoms or functional issues, then, by definition, they are not posterior tongue-ties. They must cause problems in order to justify the diagnosis and subsequent treatment— "If it ain't broke, don't fix it!"

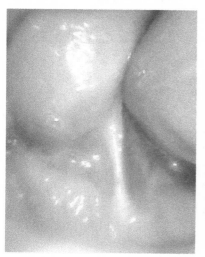 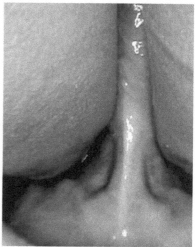

Examples of two posterior tongue-ties that were causing significant symptoms and improved after treatment.

Posterior tongue-tie was first described by Watson-Genna and Coryllos in 2004, so the concept is relatively new.[24] All tongue-ties have a submucosal component, but one kind of posterior tongue-tie is completely submucosal. The tie, or restriction, is hidden under the tissue (mucosa) lining the floor of the mouth. Upon first glance, there is no obvious or visible string of tissue, as there is with an anterior tongue-tie. Posterior ties in general consist of connective tissue that is tighter or more restrictive than normal,[25] which causes a functional issue even though it does not extend near or to the tip of the tongue.

The tongue-tie does not contain muscle itself, but it lies just over the genioglossus muscle under the tongue. When examining the tongue, the provider should position him or herself behind the baby's head, use two index fingers to elevate the tongue, and see how far up it elevates. If a tight string pops up or holds the tongue down, or you see a dimple in the middle of the tongue, these are signs of limited movement and indicate a posterior tongue-tie. If the provider runs his or her index finger under the tongue in a finger sweep maneuver (side to side), the floor of the mouth should feel smooth, soft, and spongy. If there is a feeling of tight tissue in the floor of the mouth, like a speed bump or like the finger has to jump a fence at the midline to get across to the other side, then this is a sign of a posterior tongue-tie.

If it ain't broke, don't fix it!

A posterior tongue-tie can be released with scissors by a skilled and careful provider making multiple cuts, but a laser offers better visibility and hemostasis, as we will discuss later. If a baby has all the symptoms of a tongue-tie but no visible tie, it is most likely a posterior tie. If the mother is describing all the symptoms of a tongue-tie as we discussed earlier, and the provider looks quickly and not thoroughly, a posterior tie may be missed. If the provider puts on gloves, checks from a position seated behind the baby with a headlight, and lifts up the tongue and performs the finger sweep, tighter than normal tissue will likely be evident. If symptoms exist, usually something is holding the tongue down and preventing the infant from latching properly. Many babies examined in the hospital would appear to have a posterior tongue-tie, but without symptoms and function, there is nothing to be done. This fact highlights the need to check on families one or two weeks after discharge to ensure they are able to meet their goals.

A quick word about bodywork (such as craniosacral therapy, chiropractic care, or myofascial release) would be helpful at this point. Bodywork is an important part of the team approach to the treatment of tongue-ties. It can certainly be tried first and is helpful with one-sided pain (i.e., the left breast hurts worse than the right when feeding), torticollis, or other issues, but if the nursing issues are not resolved completely, a referral to a knowledgeable release provider should be made promptly to assess for a tongue-tie. More information may be found in Chapters 24 and 25.

The Lip-Tie

While the most common presentation of restricted oral tissues is the tongue, the lip and its frena are still critical pieces of the puzzle and warrant examination. Collectively, tongue-ties, lip-ties, and buccal-ties are referred to as TOTs, or tethered oral tissues. The tissue referred to in all these cases is known as a frenum or frenulum. A restricted or tight frenum prevents normal movement of the oral tissues.

What, then, is considered to be the normal range of motion of oral soft tissue? As we have discussed, there should be a functional impact of restricted tissues along with the clinical presentation of a tie in order to justify treatment. The lip-tie can contribute to nursing difficulties for the baby and can independently make breastfeeding painful and difficult for the mother. It can contribute to a poor seal on the breast due to the inability of the upper lip to flange outward normally. In my experience, if a child only has a lip-tie, and it is released, the symptoms can and do resolve. One article also discusses the phenomenon of breastfeeding difficulties from upper lip-tie only, and in 14 babies who underwent only a lip-tie release, 78% saw improvement.[26]

The lip-tie can contribute to nursing difficulties for the baby and can independently make breastfeeding painful and difficult for the mother.

If there is a tongue-tie present as well (which is the most common presentation), then providers release both the tongue-tie and the lip-tie simultaneously. Although there is a classification system created by Dr. Kotlow (Class 1 to Class 4), the main issue when evaluating for any tie is the functional impact.[18,27] No provider, family member, or Facebook friend can diagnose a lip-tie from a photograph alone (and the same holds true for tongue-tie). In fact, most babies have what appears to be a lip-tie when the frenum is inspected visually, but only a fraction of those demonstrate significant functional impairment.

According to a study by Flinck in 1994, 93.4% of the included babies had a maxillary frenum that either inserted into the gum ridge or the palate.[28] If the baby is having nursing issues and the upper lip has a tight frenum holding it down and preventing it from flanging outward normally, there is a good chance that releasing it will help the baby. Often, a lip-tie and a tongue-tie will be present together in the same baby. According to Dr. Bobby Ghaheri, an ENT and well-known authority on tongue-tie, if there is blanching (it turns white when the lip is lifted) in the area where the frenum attaches to the tissue, if there is a dimple on the upper surface of the lip, if there is a notch in the gum tissue or bone, and/or if the lactation consultant (IBCLC) determines the baby has a latch suggesting a lip-tie, then a lip-tie may be present, and a release should be considered.[29]

If the frenum causes pain or distress to the baby when lifted, or if the tongue-tie has already been released and latching issues persist, a lip-tie may be affecting the latch as well. Some lip frena are especially thick, tight, or broad. Their shape is highly variable, but the main factor is their impact on function. If the lip won't flange outward easily, or curls under when nursing, usually the seal will be affected and the latch will be shallow. The baby

The lip-tie shape is highly variable, but the main factor is the impact on function.

29

will make clicking noises, reflux may be present, and the mother may experience discomfort.

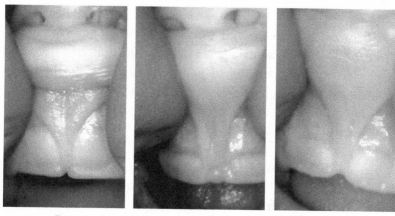

Lip-ties come in different shapes and sizes, thick or thin, and some even cause bone notching.

It is difficult to quantify which issues are related to the tongue-tie and which are related to the lip-tie because there is considerable overlap, and there are no good studies that define the distinguishing features of each disorder. We have seen mothers and infants who continue to experience persistent nursing struggles after the tongue-tie is addressed. We owe it to these mothers and babies to use the best available evidence and our clinical judgment to do something now to help them with nursing difficulties. To help the family in front of us, we create a unique plan for that individual baby using the best practice recommendations advised by the group of professionals currently treating these cases of persistent nursing difficulty. It is not a one-size-fits-all treatment.

Ideally, the lip-tie release, if needed, should happen at the same time as the tongue-tie release so the baby is not put through two different procedures. If there is a question about whether to cut or not to cut, the second correction can be performed at the one-week follow-up appointment. A recent study showed that multiple clinicians couldn't agree on the classification of the lip-tie from a photograph—whether it went all the way to the palate, or whether it stopped short.[30] The clinicians created their own grading type, which is similar to the Kotlow classification system but defines only three types: Type 1—into the area between the mucosa (cheek lining) and the gingiva (hard gum tissue); Type 2—into the mid-attached gingiva; and Type 3—into the inferior margin of the papilla (at the edge of the gum) or wrapping around to the palate. However, in the article's example photograph, Types 2 and 3 both appear to insert into the inferior ridge. They also found that the inter-rater reliability of their new scale was only 38%. The researchers concluded that because it is hard to determine the classification of each tie from a photograph, a release shouldn't be performed based on appearance alone,[30] a recommendation for which there is general agreement. You cannot diagnose a lip-tie from a photograph alone. Instead, it is more about the tactile feel of the tissue and the history reported by the mother than about how it looks. If the lip tucks in when nursing, it cannot evert properly, and the baby and/or mother may experience symptoms; in this case, a release should be discussed with the parents. The procedure carries very little risk when performed with a laser (other than minor bleeding, minor swelling, and soreness for about three days). It takes around 15 seconds when performed properly. The release technique is discussed in Chapter 7.

You cannot diagnose a lip-tie from a photograph alone.

The lip-tie comes in every conceivable shape and size. Again, most babies (more than 90%) have a frenum that extends close to or onto the palate. It can be thin or thick, fleshy or fibrous, triangular or corded, but only if it is functionally restrictive *and* the baby has nursing problems does it likely need treatment. If there are no nursing issues, no intervention is needed. We field many calls at our office from parents who are concerned that their child has a lip-tie. If upon examining that child, there is no functional restriction and/or no nursing difficulty, we do not perform the procedure. We don't treat the baby for something that may arise in the future, such as a gap between the teeth or difficulty brushing the teeth (see Chapter 21). We treat the baby based on the current issue, the best available information, the clinical exam, and the clinician's best judgment.

Some practitioners believe that a lip-tie doesn't play a significant role in nursing issues, while others have concluded that the lip-tie does, in fact, cause significant nursing issues on its own. Sometimes a lip-tie is diagnosed, but the parent elects only to release the tongue; in other cases, insurance only covers one procedure per day, and the parent chooses to wait, so only the tongue is released. This is appropriate if only one tethered tissue can be addressed because the odds are in favor of the tongue being the primary cause of nursing difficulty. The wound healing of the tongue takes about three weeks, and the lip-tie wound takes about two weeks to heal. If the parent is performing aftercare exercises or stretches (see Chapter 8) after the tongue is released, the baby can return at one week to check the healing. If symptoms still persist, the lip-tie can be released at that visit, which will not extend the overall recovery period. When the lip-tie is treated independently a week after the tongue-tie, mothers often report a significant decrease in pain, and a much better and deeper latch. It does make a difference clinically—and we often see the results immediately after the procedure before the mother leaves the office.

One Final Type: Buccal-Ties

There are no research studies mentioning the impact of buccal-ties on nursing or oral motor skills, but many providers who routinely treat restricted oral tissues acknowledge their existence and recognize that they can require intervention as well. Buccal-ties have been the subject of lectures and discussion at various professional conferences as well. There are four buccal frena in the cheek, which is what the name *buccal* (pronounced like "buckle") refers to—by the cheek. Two are in the upper arch of the mouth and two are in the lower arch.

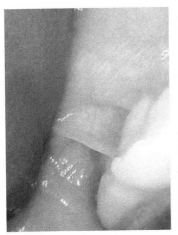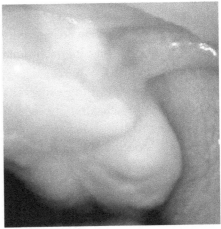

Buccal-ties can cause difficulty with cheek mobility.

The lower buccal frena do not typically seem to cause any issues. The upper buccal frena, however, can be tight, prevent the baby from moving his or her jaw or cheeks well, and contribute to nursing issues. During a first exam, after checking outside the mouth, I check inside the mouth. I first check the lip flange and upper lip frenum, and then I check the tongue movement and lingual frenum, and finally, I check the cheeks to make sure it feels smooth when rubbing a finger from front to back in the deepest part between the cheek and gums. If there is a buccal-tie, it feels tight and like a speed bump, similar to a posterior tongue-tie but in the upper cheeks. We do not charge any extra for buccal-ties in my office, and I release them far less often than the lip- or tongue-tie.

Though less common than lip- or tongue-tie, it is important to check for buccal-ties because they can restrict movement of the cheeks and lips. We have also seen a difference clinically when doing a buccal-tie release after having performed a tongue and lip release with babies still having some persistent nursing difficulties. When we released the buccal-ties, the mothers noticed a difference in the latch and experienced less pain. I have also noted that when the upper lip-tie is released and the lip still doesn't seem as mobile as it should be, the buccal-tie on one or both sides can be released with the laser in about 5 seconds per side. As a result, the upper lip will often flip up easily with more freedom and less effort.

Lactation consultants around the country are observing firsthand how these buccal-ties can inhibit the cheeks from activating properly, and seeing an immediate difference in the quality of the latch after the release because the baby can move the cheeks better and suck more effectively. Other release providers around the country are noticing these restrictive buccal frena as well and releasing them and finding similar positive results.

CHAPTER 4

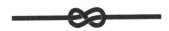

The Role of the Lactation Consultant

Lisa Lahey, RN, IBCLC

In the United States, more women are breastfeeding than in the past. Current statistics (2016) show initiation rates of 81%, but by 6 months only 22% are breastfeeding exclusively, meaning no other supplements or foods.[31] Many health organizations, including the American Academy of Pediatrics, recommend breastfeeding for 6 months, followed by complementary introduction of solid foods at 6 months and continued breastfeeding up to age 2 or as long as mutually desired.[32] The advantages of breastfeeding are the child's optimal nutrition and immunity, promoting bonding and social interactions, and helping stimulate proper growth and development of the airway and structures of the mouth and face. Breastfeeding is a foundational oral skill that is succeeded by other oral skills, such as chewing, swallowing, and speaking.

More parents desire optimal breastfeeding and breast milk for their children, but why are mothers falling short of their goals? There are multiple reasons that we as a community should strive to address and improve breastfeeding success if we want to meet our goals as a nation, such as those outlined in Healthy People 2020 (in the United States).[31] These goals include increasing the proportion of infants who are breastfed, increasing workplace lactation programs for working mothers, reducing the number of breastfed infants who receive formula within the first two days of life, and increasing the number of births in Baby Friendly hospitals.[31] We need prenatal education classes and consultations before birth to empower mothers and educate the families about the benefits and basics of breastfeeding. Next, we need hospital policies and procedures that support optimal birth and breastfeeding, such as fewer birth interventions, more and prolonged skin-to-skin contact, promoting breastfeeding early and often, avoiding unnecessary formula supplementation, and providing optimal lactation support while parents learn breastfeeding.[32] Our communities need cultures and workplaces that support and encourage breastfeeding and provide time for pumping. It is well known that the top reasons mothers decide to stop breastfeeding are poor start (i.e., difficulty successfully initiating), breast/nipple pain, latch difficulty, lack of milk supply (perceived or real), lack of support, and return to work.[33] An International Board Certified Lactation Consultant (IBCLC) can help address these concerns and optimize breastfeeding so that parents can meet their personal breastfeeding goals.

This may be the first time you have heard of an IBCLC. An IBCLC is a highly skilled allied healthcare professional who meets rigorous education and eligibility requirements, passes an independent certification examination every 5 to 10 years, and keeps current clinically with required continuing education credits. This certification differs from other lactation helpers such as peer counselors, lactation educator or counselors who have a role in support and educating families with uncomplicated breastfeeding. The education requirements, clinical competencies and scope of practice of the IBCLC focus on clinical assessment and care.

The IBCLC scope of practice and expertise includes infant and child development, nutrition, physiology, and pathology; this includes feeding behaviors at different ages and stages, introducing complementary foods, food intolerances/allergies, infant anatomy and oral anatomy, neurological challenges, muscle tone, reflexes, growth patterns/charts, and nutritional requirements. The IBCLC also provides assessment, education, and counseling on maternal lactation issues such as breast development and growth, anatomical or surgical challenges, breast infections, milk supply management, maternal nutritional status, composition of human milk, milk banking, and the impact of endocrine hormones on human lactation. The IBCLC gains knowledge and understanding about conditions such as diabetes, infertility, metabolic, hormonal, and autoimmune disorders, pharmacology, galactogogues (any substance that increases milk production), and medicinal herbs' impact on increasing breast milk supply. Unfortunately, there are some healthcare providers who rarely have the time or extra breastfeeding expertise to assess the breastfeeding mother-infant dyad together and holistically. Separating the assessment of mom and baby discounts the biological interplay and dance that happens during the act of breastfeeding where mother's issues are the baby's issues and vice versa. The IBCLC takes the time to assess both mom and baby together and plays a critical role in supporting the family as they navigate feeding transitions and challenges while ensuring that the mother is cared for emotionally as she learns her new role and how to breastfeed. Furthermore, IBCLCs are involved in psychology, sociology, research, public health, anthropology, and the dynamics of breastfeeding in the culture. IBCLCs promote, support, and advocate for the breastfeeding dyad/family in a variety of settings such as hospitals, outpatient clinics, doctor offices, and in their own private practices.

Lactation consultants use a problem-solving approach to provide clinical assessment, education, recommendations, lactation therapy, feeding plans, and referrals to other healthcare providers. IBCLCs address feeding issues that range from basic to complex. Highly skilled IBCLCs are an integral part of the tethered oral tissues (TOTs) caregiving team, working with the breastfeeding mother-baby dyad when it comes to suck dysfunction and post-frenectomy care. Suck dysfunction can be due to poor latch and positioning, uncoordinated infant reflexes and muscles, or structural and postural issues impacting function during feeding. IBCLCs have much to assess and optimize with the breastfeeding dyad, and each care plan is highly detailed and individualized. We often work with babies affected by suck dysfunction and ties, but also babies who have stopped breastfeeding directly and need help with bottle-feeding.

A primary challenge for the tethered oral tissues specialty area and for IBCLCs is a general lack of awareness among both the public and healthcare professionals of oral dysfunction and ties. There is a great need for better assessment skills, more training, and educational opportunities so that more providers are vigilant about providing appropriate care. For this reason, many IBCLCs are involved in teaching or writing books.

The next challenge is the hot button question of who can assess and diagnose. As IBCLCs, we can describe and report to the patient and medical provider what we observe and assess with the feeding assessment and oral exam. The best way to do that is by good charting, writing reports or consult notes, and communicating assessments and findings to parents and healthcare providers. We also recognize that ties can be complex and varied in signs and symptoms. I often say ties are like fingerprints, differing anatomically and functionally, so our care should respect individual needs, and we must tailor assessment, therapy, and treatment recommendations accordingly.

> *There is a great need for better assessment skills, more training, and educational opportunities so that more providers are vigilant about providing appropriate care.*

Those within the TOTs specialty area are working to develop better training for lactation consultants and medical providers so that they can be equipped to offer thorough assessments and diagnoses, full functional releases, and excellent postoperative wound care. IBCLCs who have taken time to become well versed in tongue-ties and oral function know there is a great need for well-designed research to validate the outcomes that are clearly evident to those currently practicing in this area. Until the studies are done, we will continue to offer education, communication, and a team approach that keeps patients at the center of the care equation.

Parents who seek a lactation consult often wonder why a baby can't latch or breastfeed well. IBCLCs will discuss better latch and positioning techniques and how restricted tongue mobility can be an issue that plays a key role in breastfeeding difficulty. The IBCLC understands the tongue's anatomy and physiology and the mechanics of how the tongue works during breastfeeding. The mouth opens, lips and tongue make contact with the breast and the tongue extends to grasp the areola and nipple to stabilize the breast tissue in the baby's mouth. Next, the cupping of the tongue around the nipple creates a seal, the tongue elevates and presses against the palate and the lower jaw drops to create the necessary vacuum to extract milk.[12] The mid to posterior tongue controls the movement of the fluid for good swallowing and optimal airway protection, as the palate and tongue work to close off the nasopharyngeal space during the suck, swallow, breathe sequence. The tongue also helps to shape and form the palate and dental arch and provides feedback to the autonomic nervous system to be regulated.

The IBCLC Must Assess with Finesse

Let's discuss how an IBCLC assesses feeding and oral function. When IBCLCs first meet a mother in person or by phone, we utilize active listening skills to learn about the concerns and feeding problems, noting both maternal and infant symptoms. Next, we ask in-depth questions to ensure we have a full medical and feeding history. Intake interviews often take 1 hour or more and include prenatal, pregnancy, and birth history. We ask about prior breastfeeding experiences, maternal diet, medications, and any chronic or current health issues of mom or baby. We discuss feeding routines and patterns, the infant's urine and stool counts, baby's weight gain and growth, personal breastfeeding goals, and the support system of the dyad. The IBCLC sets up an appointment to consult in the home, office, or outpatient setting, where we observe the baby feeding, offer a maternal breast exam, assist with latch and positioning, assess milk transfer by weighing the baby before and after feeding on an accurate and highly sensitive digital scale, perform an oral suck exam on our gloved finger to evaluate the suck, and assess oral motor skills of the tongue, cheeks, lips, palate, and jaws.

A proper functional exam for ties starts with the feeding assessment. How does the baby latch and position at the breast? Does the mother have to make several adjustments or make heroic efforts to make the feeding work? The IBCLC will assess for wide gape, flanged lips, seal, and tongue extension past the lower gum ridge to locate and cup the nipple while maintaining suction. The cheeks should appear round and full, not hollow or dimpling. The jaw movements are smooth and rhythmic to allow for good suck, swallow, and breathing patterns. The sucking pattern should be organized with adequate sucking bursts and swallows heard every 1 to 3 sucks that are quiet but remain vigorous while breast milk is released and transferred. Baby should remain alert and relaxed at the breast and have enough stamina throughout the feeding until releasing the breast, satisfied and milk drunk. During this time we observe the mother to assess comfort and her ability to nurse without pain. We ask her to describe what the latch and sucking feels like and don't rely only on what a latch looks like from the outside view.

Red flags that often arise with feeding typically fall into one of two types: low-tone sucking and high-tone sucking. Babies with low-tone sucking will root frantically, but can't latch or latch poorly. After many attempts, the baby will often slip off or maintain only light flutter suction and may not feed through multiple letdowns. The low-tone sucking baby falls asleep at the breast when exerting too great of an effort or the baby decides to shut down before sufficient milk is removed. The baby often likes to graze at the breast and feeds softly and often. Mom is rarely sore, and these babies are at risk for slow or no weight gain. Parents can be fooled because the baby feeds often and painlessly. Other babies will respond with high tone and increased sucking effort to get the milk any way they can, so they bite or clamp down to get milk to flow, or suck harder with tight lips and increased cheek activity. The baby with a high-tone suck often causes much pain and damage to the nipples due to improper balance or forces of the lip and cheeks. When the baby releases the nipple, there can be a white line/crease mark, lipstick-shaped nipple, a vasospasm (sudden painful constriction of a blood vessel) skin response, and, with repeated trauma every few hours, the nipple tissue becomes sore and wounded with cracks, blisters, blebs, or bleeding.

Babies with submucosal tongue-ties often have a lot of difficulties lifting the mid-tongue and cupping the lateral borders of the tongue, making for a disorganized swallow. These babies may produce clicking or smacking sounds while they feed in addition to gulping, coughing, gagging, and choking noises. Babies should eat without much noise at all, and these babies cannot handle the flow of milk well, often taking in large amounts of air and presenting with aerophagia and reflux. The mothers often report oversupply and overactive milk letdown. The baby with a posterior tie often rejects the idea of pacifiers or taking breast milk by bottle. My theory is that the mother's breasts and body know the suck is suboptimal and, coupled with frequent overstimulation, the breast dumps milk fast and furiously. The baby will exhibit behaviors like arching the back, tightly straining the upper body, and undergoing a stiffness resembling military posture. The baby struggles to maintain the airway while feeding and can have difficulty protecting the airway. As a result, the baby comes off the breast, thereby breaking suction, and doesn't seem to rest and digest. Often a gassy or fussy baby needs to remain upright or be walked around for extended periods after a feeding. The mom will say the baby hates to breastfeed or only breastfeeds when in a certain position, such as lying down, or when drowsy or asleep. I also have observed that these are the babies that are at risk for stopping breastfeeding abruptly and for oral aversion. They also typically need more support before and after frenectomy to achieve optimal suck and feeding.

Our goal as IBCLCs is to support breastfeeding while making sure the baby is optimally fed and mom's milk supply is increased or protected until the issues resolve and/or a frenectomy is performed (if needed). Depending on the circumstances, we may recommend a nipple shield and/or supplementation during feeding by offering mom's milk, donor milk, or formula by tube at the breast, utilizing a lactation aid or supplemental nursing system (SNS).

IBCLC TOTs Exam

IBCLCs often use a functional assessment tool to guide their assessment of ties. The three best validated tools currently available are the Hazelbaker Assessment Tool for Lingual Frenulum Function (HATLFF),[34] the Frenotomy Decision Rule for Breastfeeding Infants (FDRBI) by Dobrich,[35] and the Martinelli Lingual Frenulum Protocol.[36]

These tools can assist in the evaluation of appearance and function, but they each have limitations, so the IBCLC uses his or her combined clinical experience and differential assessment skills to help get a full picture of the oral exam. IBCLCs may begin by letting the baby suck on a finger. They may start by tapping lightly on the baby's lips, waiting for the finger to go (pad side up) to the hard and soft palate junction to assess how strong or weak suction is, where the tongue movements originate, and how the tongue cups, lateralizes, lifts, extends, or retracts. We take note of the shape and arch of the palate, the length of the palate, the gag reflex, and the suck quality for tone, strength, rhythm, and cupping. We may use a curved syringe to add milk during a digital suck exam to evaluate the baby's response and compare the quality of the suck with and without a fluid bolus. The Murphy maneuver (named after Dr. Jim Murphy, a pediatrician, breastfeeding medicine specialist, and IBCLC) is also performed during the suck exam by using the first finger to gently sweep under the tongue, left and right, to assess for a string of tissue that is tight or raised, preventing a smooth sweep across the floor of the mouth.

Next, we assess other areas that can impact the suck, swallow, breathing pattern, and the ability to latch and position with ease, such as the baby's body posture. Babies that have conditions like torticollis, plagiocephaly, facial asymmetries, or postural strains can be uncomfortable, making it harder to latch, position, and feed well. An IBCLC holds the baby or child on a flat surface to look at his or her side-lying, prone, and supine positions. We observe the overall body, posture, and tone during movement, which may be soft, firm, tense, relaxed, or at ease. How do the neck, shoulders, arms, legs, and hips move and respond to touch and movement? Extension and flexion are analyzed as we play with the baby. Does the baby's body curve or stay in straight alignment? Next, we note the face, eyes, and jaws/chin for symmetry. We assess the shape of the head—front, back, sides, fontanels, and cranial ridges—taking notes about abnormalities such as odd-shaped, raised, or flattened areas. For example, a baby who shows a head turn preference or tension on the left side of the neck may latch easily to the right breast but not latch comfortably to the left breast. In this case, manual therapy or bodywork, such as myofascial or craniosacral therapy by a trained professional (osteopath, chiropractor, PT, OT, LMT, SLP, or RN), may be employed to help relax tight muscles that may be affecting feeding. While this may help resolve feeding issues for some babies, a lack of response leads to concluding that the ties are contributing to dysfunctional feeding and the noted fascial strains. If that happens, it is time to refer for frenectomy.

Mouth Exam for TOTs

The assessor, usually an IBCLC, will place the baby in the proper knee-to-knee position or place the baby flat on his or her back on an exam table, with the baby's head near the assessor and toes pointing away. The assessor stands or sits behind the baby's head just as a dentist would to perform an exam. We cradle the baby's head between the palms of our hands and, using both first fingers, pull the upper lip up toward the nose. We note any tension or difficulty lifting the lip, look for the lip to flange up easily to the nostrils, assess for the upper lip to dip down or bunch like an accordion near the philtrum, assess whether the lip-tie is thick or thin, and determine where the frenum attaches on the gum ridge. Next, we look for blanching and notching on the upper alveolar gum ridge. We also sweep a finger over the upper gum ridge to assess for buccal-ties. A buccal-tie that stops a gentle finger sweep, that is attached low to the gum ridge or beyond the mucogingival line, or that causes blanching on the gums warrants further assessment of symptoms with lip tension and seal while feeding.

To evaluate the tongue or lingual restriction, the assessor uses both index fingers to get under the tongue and push down into the floor of mouth, gently lifting up the tongue as high as possible and back toward the throat, holding the middle fingers on the jaw to stabilize the tongue lift assessment. We note the tension and elasticity, length of a tie if present and where it attaches, and whether the tie is thick or thin. We palpate the lingual frenum for tension, look for blanching, examine the appearance of the tongue tip and describe it as heart-shaped or indented, and note whether the tongue is squared off or coated white. The assessor takes time to look at the hard and soft palate. We often take photos of the ties or have parents take photos of ties and help them set up the smartphone or camera in an ideal position and angle, using the flash to capture the ties for their records.

The IBCLC will next effectively communicate and explain to the parents the findings of the assessment and how function and feeding are being impacted. We often share photos, parent-friendly educational articles, or handouts we have made that are tailored to issues that may need further explanation or educational reinforcement. An important role that the IBCLC performs is to provide anticipatory guidance and education about what to expect during and after frenectomy and other tie releases. We explain how the procedure is performed as well as the relevant benefits and risks. We then discuss what to expect with healing and wound care, offering comfort techniques and common homeopathic or conventional medications that may be used for discomfort, along with tips for recovery and successful rehabilitation.

The lactation consultant reviews pre-frenectomy oral exercises, wound aftercare instructions, and the care plan that is individualized to the dyad for addressing problems such as increasing weight gain and supply prior to referring for the frenectomy. The consult note and feeding plan are then provided to the parents and the baby's medical doctor, and a referral for bodywork and/or a frenectomy provider is given. Follow-up appointments are set up to review feeding progress, oral exercises, post-frenectomy aftercare, and emotional support during healing. Parents often need reminding that frenectomy is often not a quick fix and that ties have been restricting function and feeding for an extended period of time. Therefore, patience, time, and effort through therapy are required for successful oral rehabilitation in which the baby learns how to move his or her tongue and lips in a whole new way. Post-revision, the baby will need modification of the mother's technique with latch and feeding. She may need to be taught new techniques such as how to latch without a nipple shield, how to select a nursing position that no longer requires her to compensate, and how to perform effective breast shaping and compressions. The oral exercises and suck training help to rehabilitate the movement and function of the tongue, jaw, lips, and cheeks. Clearly, IBCLCs who have taken extra training and specialize in complex feeding and oral rehabilitation are able to offer considerable support and assistance to help the dyad successfully optimize a new latch, stabilize feeding behaviors, and enhance nursing skills post frenectomy, and several appointments may be needed to review oral exercises and feeding skills to optimize function.

Patience, time, and effort through therapy are required for successful oral rehabilitation.

If the baby is still struggling 1 to 2 weeks after the frenectomy, the IBCLC will suggest a follow-up visit to teach specific suck training and oral exercises based on any issues identified during the reassessment. Showing parents how to do tummy time, infant massage, reflex integration, and baby play activities help to strengthen the baby's neck, shoulders, and other muscles that support effective feeding. Coordination with bodywork professionals is encouraged to further support optimal rehabilitation (see Chapter 25 for more information).

Assessment of Oral Tissues in Older Babies to Toddlers

The IBCLC works not only with infants but with older babies and toddlers that are continuing to breastfeed, transition to solid foods, or may be starting the process of weaning. Parents reach out for education and support to the IBCLC in all of these circumstances and more. IBCLCs are knowledgeable about symptoms that the older baby may have, such as ongoing weight or feeding issues, difficulty transitioning to solid foods (with symptoms such as texture aversions, choking, gagging, vomiting, pocketing food or slow eating), delayed speech or difficulty speaking, and dental abnormalities. With any of these symptoms, an IBCLC will notify the pediatrician and then refer to speech or occupational therapy. The feeding team including the IBCLC subsequently discusses and makes recommendations for optimizing breastfeeding, solid food eating, and for frenectomy as needed if the symptoms point to ties and functional feeding issues.

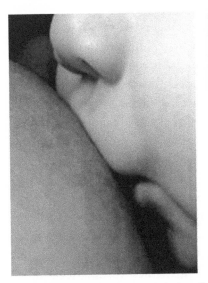 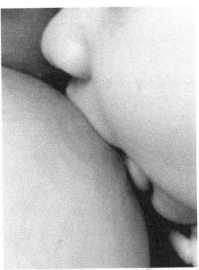

*Baby's shallow latch before (left), and after the tongue- and
lip-tie release (right) on the same day.
Notice the mouth is open wider and baby's lips are less pursed.*

Anticipatory Guidance with Aftercare

If restrictive ties are present and the baby is being referred for further evaluation, it is best to discuss and teach the wound care lifts of the tongue and lip at the first consult. The consultant will model the care and interaction parents will need with post-frenectomy stretches or lifts and can guide best ways to position their fingers inside the baby's mouth for oral rehabilitation exercises and aftercare.

Next, parents are encouraged to practice twice a day before the frenectomy and prior to an actual wound being present. Doing this builds the parents' confidence, which in turn helps the child become more familiar with the process of aftercare and suck training; additionally, these oral exercises start to fire and wire the muscles to help overall tone and strength.

Finally, a care plan for comfort and post-procedure discomfort is discussed. Parents need a checklist of what to purchase, such as homeopathics, teething drops, and/or pain medicines ahead of time. We discuss with parents that being available a few days to a week post-frenectomy to care for baby will help optimize comfort. Holding the baby more than usual, increasing skin-to-skin time, giving the baby warm baths, and increasing baby's attempt at breast are all interventions to consider. Parents should recognize that the first 7 to 10 days post-frenectomy can be challenging because of discomfort, frequent aftercare lifts, and follow-up care appointments to various providers. Parents are encouraged to call or schedule a follow-up visit with the IBCLC 2 to 5 days post-frenectomy, 2 weeks post-frenectomy, and then as needed, depending on the age of the baby and stage of the feeding progress. Ideally, 2 to 6 follow-up appointments with the IBCLC will get feeding back on track. IBCLC follow-up appointments focus on providing parents reassurance of normal healing, optimizing new feeding techniques, working through feeding care plan items such as low milk supply, reviewing oral exercises, and offering emotional support for parents. Parents often have many questions and begin to doubt the procedure was effective or valuable during this time of transition and healing. We can encourage and point out where progress is being made and continue to teach parents what they can do to help the child on the road to recovery. Sometimes parents want to talk to other parents whose children have experienced frenectomy, so the IBCLC can connect parents with others who have experienced similar issues, or recommend attending a support group, either in person or online.

> *Holding the baby more than usual, increasing skin-to-skin time, giving the baby warm baths, and increasing baby's attempt at breast are all interventions to consider.*

IBCLC Challenges to Care

Oftentimes, IBCLCs meet dyads for whom the opportunity to recover the milk supply fully has passed, or the baby has been away from direct or frequent breastfeeding for many months and is now either partially breastfeeding or bottle-feeding exclusively. In these cases, the IBCLC will work to praise the mother's efforts and encourage mom that her quantity of milk, even when combined with formula, still benefits the child's growth and immune system. Babies that are bottle-fed can struggle with sucking skills, too; sometimes we see babies demonstrate fussy and frustrated behaviors while taking the bottle, dribbling or leaking milk while bottle-feeding, and taking 30 minutes or more to finish a bottle, in which case the baby is expending too much energy, which may lead to poor weight gain or bottle refusal.

We do our best to help optimize milk supply, demonstrate better ways to bottle-feed, and discuss relactation efforts if possible. Parents grieve the loss of breastfeeding when ties impact early feeding, but the IBCLC can plant the seeds for breastfeeding success for the next child they have by encouraging parents to contact the lactation consultant within the first week after the next birth. Working with feeding challenges has many highs and lows, but the rewards are thrilling when parents share success stories and persevere until their babies progress to better feeding and developmental paths.

CHAPTER 5

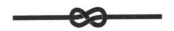

The Release Provider's Assessment

The young infant with a tongue-tie is perhaps the most challenging patient with a tongue-tie to treat because timing is critical, and all players on the treatment team need to be connected and on the same page. Patients of all ages face unique challenges with recovery and need to learn correct muscle coordination and/or unlearn compensatory muscle use in order to achieve normal function of the tongue. Babies are no different, and many require significant assistance during rehabilitation.

Treating a baby should start in the hospital, with an exam after birth. Babies are assessed for a number of potential problems at birth, and in some countries, such as Brazil, there is legislation that helps. Brazil has a frenum inspection law that requires the free evaluation of the lingual frenum in all infants by a speech-language pathologist, who is looking for restrictions such as tongue-tie.[37,38] This type of legislation would be helpful in many countries, including the United States, and support for it is growing. The key is to ensure that those inspecting the baby's mouth and oral tissues know what to look for and are properly trained in methods to accurately assess and treat any noted restrictions.

Just as babies are examined for numerous other congenital abnormalities, a tongue-tie assessment should be done at birth by a provider who has received recent continuing education on assessing for the full spectrum of tongue-ties. The findings, if any, should be discussed with the lactation consultant (IBCLC), who would make a separate evaluation and assess all aspects of the breastfeeding relationship. The IBCLC should assess the latch, evaluate the mother feeding the baby, ask follow-up questions, counsel, and inspect the mouth for a tongue-tie or lip-tie, as discussed in detail in the previous chapter. Although the lactation consultant cannot officially diagnose tethered tissues, the IBCLC's scope of practice does support the assessment of infant oral tissues, which is key to determining whether there is a functional issue. If there is a suspicion of a tongue- and/or lip-tie, the IBCLC should make a referral to an appropriate provider for further evaluation of any tied tissue and treatment if necessary.

Lactation consultants are advocates for the family, and the hospital and attending physicians should give them the ability to work within their scope of practice. The lactation consultants should provide education and guidance to the families regarding tongue-ties. Often with a posterior tongue-tie, initially there are not many symptoms that are different from those of a non-tongue-tied baby attempting to latch for the first time. There can be difficulty latching, initial discomfort, and some fussiness, and all of that can be considered normal. The hospital-based IBCLC, however, should counsel the family that if the breastfeeding becomes worse or other problems arise, they should return for an evaluation with the IBCLC or seek out a tongue-tie-savvy provider. The hospital should ensure that parents know they can return to the lactation consultant, find an IBCLC in private practice, or attend a community breastfeeding support group if nursing challenges persist after the new family arrives at home. An IBCLC is the quarterback of the nursing team, visiting with the mother and baby more often than other providers (either at

The hospital should ensure that parents know they can return to the lactation consultant if nursing challenges persist after the new family arrives at home.

home, in a support group, or at a clinic), and guiding nursing dyads during the crucial postpartum period and beyond.

Once a tongue-tie is identified, a referral should be made to a knowledgeable provider. After our twin girls were diagnosed and treated with tongue-tie and experienced great improvement, I read countless articles, watched videos, attended conferences, read books, and conversed with release providers across the country to learn as much as possible about this topic. Significant self-study and future study must occur to begin treating infants. There are many different types of providers involved in the care of these tongue-tied babies. It takes a team of people to care for the mother and baby properly, as evidenced by the professionals contributing to this book.

As mentioned previously, the IBCLC may be the first one to identify an issue in the breastfeeding relationship, and her expertise goes far beyond merely assessing the latch or helping with positioning—as I learned firsthand with our girls. The act of breastfeeding is difficult for some babies, which surprises some mothers and healthcare providers because they expect it to come naturally and instinctively. Again, the IBCLC should refer the family to other healthcare providers if specialized care is needed. Then the family should return to the IBCLC for follow-up visits and support after a release is performed, as described in Chapter 4.

Once it is determined that a struggling breastfeeding dyad needs evaluation for possible surgery, the tongue-tie release provider is consulted. This person can be a physician, such as a pediatrician, neonatologist or otolaryngologist (ENT surgeon), a general or pediatric dentist, a periodontist, an oral surgeon, a nurse practitioner, or another healthcare provider with adequate training and licensing to perform the procedure. Many types of providers are capable of doing the procedure correctly, giving the patient a full and

The tool (laser, scissors, scalpel) selected for performance of the procedure is less important than the ability of the provider to achieve a full functional release.

functional release, and offering excellent follow-up. Likewise, the tool (laser, scissors, scalpel) selected for performance of the procedure is less important than the ability of the provider to achieve a full functional release. If a patient reports a "snip" or a "clip" was done, there is a chance it was not enough, because providers with more experience in the field typically use terms such as *tongue-tie release* or *tongue-tie revision*.

A provider performing release surgeries should be knowledgeable about both anterior and posterior tongue-ties, lip-ties, the consequences of an untreated tie throughout the lifespan of the patient, and the aftercare exercises needed. The provider should perform a full exam, answer the parents' questions, obtain informed consent for the procedure, and explain all the risks, benefits, and treatment alternatives to the parents. In some cases, parents aren't informed that their baby has had his or her frenum clipped in the hospital until *after* it is done. Many times, this type of release proves to be incomplete (as well as unethical). The provider should focus on getting a proper release with multiple small follow-up cuts utilizing proper illumination, magnification, and stabilization. It should be an extraordinarily rare case that a baby would need to be put to sleep under general anesthesia to complete the procedure. This recommendation is because the risks of general anesthesia, both at the time of the procedure and in the future, outweigh the benefits. If the procedure can be performed safely with minimal stress or discomfort to the child, then the benefits of in-office frenectomy far outweigh the risks and expense of sedation or anesthesia in a hospital setting.

> *The scissors provider should focus on getting a proper release with multiple small follow-up cuts utilizing proper illumination, magnification, and stabilization.*

The Food and Drug Administration (FDA) recently came out with new warnings against using sedatives and general anesthetics in children younger than three years of age, and animal models have shown brain cell death and other ill effects to a child's development after exposure to these medications.[39] The FDA recommends that general anesthetics be used for significant surgeries that cannot be delayed, such as congenital heart defects, cleft palate, etc. The effects of the general anesthesia medications and gases on the developing brain have not been fully studied, and there is cause for concern when sedating or putting a child to sleep if an alternative exists.[40]

The use of anesthesia always demands calculations of risk vs. benefit. If a child has a significant heart condition, general anesthesia is required during the repair. For children with a mouthful of dental decay and infection, pediatric dentists utilize general anesthesia in outpatient surgery centers to facilitate treatment of young children. This practice minimizes psychological trauma and allows treatments to be completed efficiently and with higher quality than what can be achieved in a conscious young child who is very anxious. However, a procedure like a frenectomy that can be performed safely in office does not require general anesthesia. Occasionally providers may elect to offer it, but it should only very rarely be necessary since the procedure is typically not much more traumatizing than a routine immunization, and certainly much less involved than circumcision.

Frenectomy can be performed safely in office and does not normally require general anesthesia.

The knowledge to treat these tethered tissues well must be sought out by providers because it is not typically taught in detail in medical school or residency. And if it is taught during training, it is often outdated and incorrect. The release provider should have completed some continuing-education courses related to tongue-ties in the last few years because the methods and ideas about how best to treat tongue-tie are evolving rapidly. A qualified provider can be recognized by his or her willingness to work alongside other team members, such as IBCLCs, to answer questions, show examples of past cases performed under his or her care, and demonstrate up-to-date credentials and continuing education completion related to tethered oral tissues.

The Healthcare Provider's Exam

A provider can be anyone who is interacting with the baby, such as a pediatrician, lactation consultant, speech-language pathologist (SLP), occupational therapist (OT), feeding specialist, or the release provider, as discussed previously. The provider should first take a medical history and have the mother fill out a questionnaire that includes all relevant issues that could be related to the baby's tongue-tie (see Appendix). The mother may not realize that spitting up, reflux, thrush, mastitis, and not being able to hold a pacifier in the mouth can be related to a tongue-tie. After mom fills out the questionnaire, the baby must be taken out of the car seat and out of the mother's arms and placed on an exam table, a dental chair, or a knee-to-knee board that fits on the laps of the mom and provider so mom can hold and see the baby while the provider visualizes the oral cavity.

The best position to evaluate for a tie is typically from above the baby as he or she is lying down, but some providers prefer to examine from below. It is possible to miss a tongue-tie that is not as obvious (such as a posterior tie) if the baby is examined from below because the lower gum pad can block the line of sight for this area.

The provider should check for the tongue-tie with two index fingers and push down on either side of the frenum and try to elevate the tongue. If the tongue does not elevate easily, there could be a restriction. Even if the baby can stick out the tongue, this does not mean there is no tongue-tie. Sometimes it is obvious from across the room that the tie goes all the way to the tip of the tongue. Other times it is more subtle and requires a closer look to see it. Either way, a full exam is warranted to make sure nothing that could complicate feeding is missed.

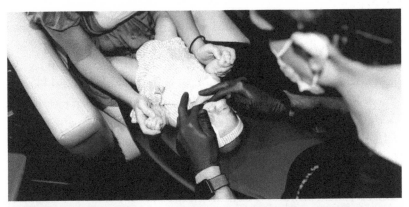

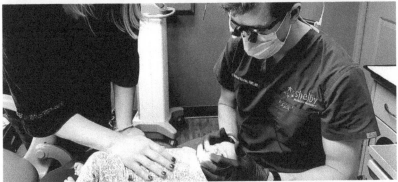

*Examining the baby on a special lap board (top) or chair (bottom)
from behind with magnification and illumination.*

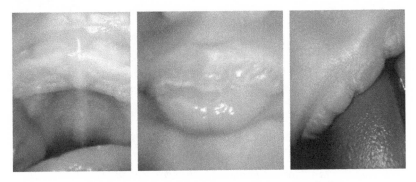

High-arched palate and sucking blisters on a baby.

Another good test is called the Murphy maneuver, as mentioned in Chapter 4. It consists of running an index finger back and forth under the tongue in the floor of the mouth. The tissues under the tongue should feel smooth, soft, and spongy. It should not feel like the finger has to jump a fence or go over a speed bump when passing the middle area under the tongue (see photo of two symptomatic ties that felt like a fence and speed bump). The palate should not be high or look like a cave, and should be more of a flat, broad, U shape. The tongue molds the palate when nursing and resting against the palate, so if the tongue is held down by a tight frenum, the palate will not be flat and broad but rather high and arched. The molding process happens in utero as well, when the baby swallows amniotic fluid and the tongue rests on the palate. A baby typically begins swallowing at 20 weeks in utero. If this swallowing pattern is abnormal, and the tongue does not touch the palate when swallowing and does not rest on the palate, babies are likely to be born with a high-arched palate. This sign often points to some kind of tongue restriction.

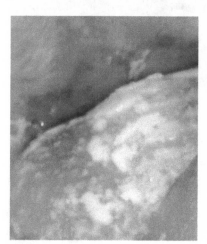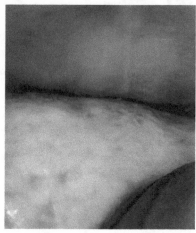

Thrush (left) in a newborn is chunky and usually occurs on the cheeks, palate, and tongue. The white-coated tongue caused by a tongue-tie (right) is smooth and white and localized to the back portion of the tongue. The latter condition does not require treatment and often disappears within a few weeks of a release.

Many tied babies have a white coating on the tongue that is often misdiagnosed as thrush. This white coating (also called milk tongue) is because the tongue does not contact the palate while resting (low tongue posture), and the milk is not scraped off naturally. A baby's tongue, like an adult's, should rest on the palate when not in use. These babies do not need thrush medication, and if white coating is seen only on the tongue, the provider should have a high degree of suspicion for a tongue restriction. Another telltale sign in tied babies is sucking blisters or calluses on the lips. These indicate a dysfunctional suck that relies on the lips to create a vacuum instead of the tongue. Additionally, babies who hiccup excessively (or hiccuped often in utero) may be more likely to have oral ties due to nerve issues, such as the vagus nerve and the phrenic nerve which innervates the diaphragm. This signals immaturity and dysregulation of the nervous system.

The ability to stick out the tongue does not rule out a tongue-tie.

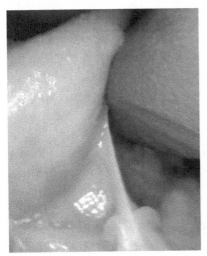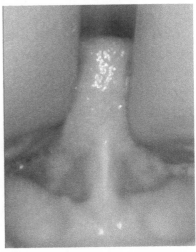

Examples of what would feel like a "fence" upon finger sweep (left), and "speed bump" (right).

A restricted tongue can lead to dental and airway issues throughout life, because the palate is the floor of the nasal cavity (see Chapter 20). The upper lip should be lifted to make sure that it is not being held down by a restricted frenum. The upper lip frenum should not blanch (turn white) or cause discomfort to the child when it is lifted up. Lip-ties can present in a variety of ways, and should be ruled out by history and examination. An experienced provider can and should assess all of the lip, tongue, and buccal areas.

Other Team Members

Often a baby who has a tongue-tie can have other problems that may need the professional help of a bodyworker, such as a physical therapist, occupational therapist, chiropractor, craniosacral therapist, or other professional who has experience and training in safely working with babies. Torticollis, for example, is a common condition from a neck muscle that is too tight on one side and can cause the head to prefer to turn to one side. This condition can cause the baby to nurse better on one side or prefer one breast over the other. If this is the case, it is good to have an evaluation by a professional who has the proper training to work with babies with torticollis and experience working with babies with restricted frenums like tongue- and lip-tie.

Sometimes a baby will need additional help feeding, and a speech therapist, feeding specialist, or occupational therapist might be consulted. Any issues with swallowing or complex medical conditions such as cleft palate would likely need the help of additional multidisciplinary team members. Typically, the release provider or lactation consultant will have a list of specialists who have assisted previous tongue-tied patients with good success. Another place to find referrals is on location-specific tongue-tie support pages on Facebook or other social media platforms.

CHAPTER 6

———— ∞ ————

Compassionate Care

Parents frequently report that they feel their obstetrician, pediatrician, or dentist has demonstrated a lack of understanding, compassion, or both, once they express concern that their child may have a tongue-tie. Often the providers encourage a mother to give the baby formula if breastfeeding is proving difficult. Even if this is said gently, with the best of intentions, mothers may not appreciate this suggestion. The mother may not have had her birth plan go the way she wanted, but at least feeding her child should come naturally and without complications, or so she thinks.

My own wife felt this way. We were hoping for a birth process that did not require much medical intervention, but when we found out that we had twins coming and one of our girls was in the breech position, we had to accept that we would need a Cesarean delivery. The procedure went well, and the babies were healthy, but nursing proved to be a monumental struggle from day one. We didn't know it at the time, but we later discovered that both girls had tongue- and lip-ties. Even though pediatricians, nurses, and lactation consultants examined them in the hospital, tongue- and lip-ties were never recognized. We were advised to supplement our girls with formula before leaving the hospital, which was not in accordance with our desires. Formula is a viable solution for some mothers, and there should not be any embarrassment or shame about using it if that is what a mother desires or decides is best. If a mother wishes to exclusively breastfeed her child, however, those wishes should be respected and every possible action should be taken to make the breastfeeding relationship successful.

Some mothers relate stories of providers who downplay or minimize the pain they experience during nursing and tell them it will go away in time, that their nipples will toughen up and build calluses. They hear the oft-repeated phrase: "That's just the way it is for some mothers." Severe pain during nursing, however, should not automatically be accepted or ignored. If a mother has pain of 9 on a 0-to-10 scale, something could be wrong. If a patient tells a physician during an office visit that she is having 9 out of 10 pain in a body part, the physician will immediately evaluate the patient to learn more about the symptom.

Significant pain is not normal; rather, it is a sign that something is not right, and should be investigated.

Now that we know more about breastfeeding challenges, it is time for physicians to learn to take a similar approach with mothers and painful nursing. Physicians need to start by truly listening to the mothers' concerns and being ready to refer them to knowledgeable providers like IBCLCs for evaluation.

It seems like a basic question, but it is important to pause and consider what it means for practitioners to treat patients compassionately. One of the most important skills a provider can learn is to listen to patients actively with the intent of learning the patient's story. Sometimes it is therapeutic for a patient simply to be heard and to be able to tell her story. It also enhances the patient's experience and relieves some of the basic stress associated with any healthcare encounter.

One of the easiest ways to begin to consciously listen better to patients is to give the patient one full minute to talk before saying anything at all to them. It can be surprising how long a full minute can take. The advent of electronic medical records has exacerbated the provider-patient listening gap, because the computer demands so many boxes are checked and blanks filled in.[41] Trying to meet patients where they are and understand their struggles should be the foremost goal of any interaction between a provider and patient. Having patient-centered interactions and making direct eye contact with the patient and the family members can lead to trust and real communication. Giving patients full attention also facilitates empathy and compassion. Allowing adequate time in the schedule to perform a detailed history and exam is a critical requirement of excellent care. Providers who have not yet had personal experience with tongue-ties can read the stories related here as well as elsewhere to get a jumpstart on understanding the struggles and exhaustion faced by families affected by this condition.

Providers who are people of faith often find that offering to pray with their patients is an excellent way to demonstrate compassion. Families almost always happily accept offers to pray with them, and find prayers calming in the stressful situations in which the parents and children find themselves. Prayers for healing for the child, for guidance and wisdom for the surgery, for a great nursing relationship for mom and baby, for peace for mom and dad, and for minimal discomfort for the baby are appropriate. Many families mention how much it means to them when their doctor prays with them before a procedure. It may well be the most memorable moment of a family's entire experience.

> *Many families mention how much it means to them when their doctor prays with them before a procedure.*

CHAPTER 7

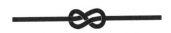

Releasing a Tongue-Tie

After the child is assessed and a thorough history points to the need to release the tongue-tie, lip-tie, and/or buccal-ties, the provider has a few different options. This chapter examines these options in depth to help parents and other team members (non-release providers) know the steps involved in treatment. This section is not intended to be used to teach someone who has never performed the procedure to go and do so. Providers interested in acquiring skill in this area should seek additional training: read books, attend continuing-education conferences, attain certifications, and shadow providers who are actively and regularly correcting the conditions. There is no substitute for hands-on experience and practice when learning to perform any surgical technique. Patient safety must always be the first concern. As with any other surgery, for a quality release, the practitioner must be both careful and methodical.

For a quality release, the practitioner must be both careful and methodical.

Options

Historically, a release of the tongue was performed by a midwife with a sharp fingernail, but today we have better options. Formerly, the primary way a release was performed was with scissors. That worked, but could be messy, and a full release could be difficult to achieve. As soon as the tissue was cut, it began to bleed, and follow-up cuts were difficult to perform with the surgical field obscured. Some providers still use scissors, but follow-up of such patients reveals a wide range of results. Some patients will have only a small nick in the still large frenum, but in some cases, the surgeon achieves a nice diamond-shaped wound under the tongue.

Interestingly, frenotomy is successfully completed (achieving a diamond shape) more often in Europe than in the United States, but it varies by practitioner. Often it is somewhere in between, meaning the practitioner clipped the frenum and left a small vertical line-shaped wound, so the anterior tongue-tie has been released, but the posterior component of the tongue-tie still exists. This incomplete release leaves a thick band of tissue that still holds the tongue in a downward position and limits mobility for nursing, speech, and/or feeding. This thick band does not go away over time, and many adults who were clipped with scissors in infancy continue to experience restrictions of their tongues that cause functional issues throughout their lives (see Chapter 29).

The incomplete release leaves a thick band of tissue that still holds the tongue in a downward position and limits mobility for nursing, speech, and/or feeding.

Dr. Bobby Ghaheri describes a tongue-tie as a sailboat. Sometimes a provider takes care of the apparent sail, but fails to release the substantial thick tissue behind the sail, analogous to a mast. He states that all anterior tongue-ties have a posterior mast component, meaning that all tongue-ties are inherently posterior ties and some also have an anterior thin membrane. If only the thin membrane is removed, the thick posterior part remains. He argues that the tool used doesn't matter as much as achieving a full release. The sailboat is a helpful analogy, and it explains why sometimes a release works and sometimes it doesn't. Some babies just need a small amount of extra freedom in their tongue mobility to breastfeed efficiently. Other babies, however, need the whole thing released. It is impossible to know which ones will see benefit from having only the anterior portion clipped, so it is best to do a complete release the first time on every patient with a symptomatic restriction.

All tongue-ties, anterior and posterior have a posterior component that must be released as well.
– Bobby Ghaheri, MD

A complete release of a tongue-tie can be compared with the surgery for syndactyly, which was discussed earlier in this book. If two webbed fingers are separated only to the first knuckle, the child might have some functional improvement; but to truly give the child the best chance of normal use of the fingers, a full release should be the goal. We don't know if the child is going to be a concert pianist, but no one debates whether the fingers should be cut halfway or fully. It should be the same with the tongue. It is best to release the whole tongue properly and fully, which is achieved with a variety of methods and proper training. No child should have to compensate for months, years, or decades, when normal mobility and function can be so easily attained.

Typically, with scissors a full release would involve using a hemostat to clamp the blood vessels in the frenum by squeezing it tightly, then making a cut in the middle of the frenum and additional smaller cuts on either side, or using what's known as blunt dissection until a diamond-shaped window opens up where the frenum used to be. What is often done during a scissors release is just one cut, which is insufficient. Follow-up cuts are the step that is most commonly left out.

What is often done during a scissors release is just one cut, which is insufficient.

The reason the wound is a diamond shape is that the frenum is triangular, and when a triangular prism is cut through, the top and bottom flip out, forming a diamond. There is no need to create a diamond because this is the natural shape the tissue takes when a sufficiently deep horizontal cut through the frenum is made. When using scissors, these smaller follow-up cuts to release tension on the lateral edges are made more difficult because of the bleeding that occurs after the first cut. The follow-up cuts remove mucosa and fascia or connective tissue, not muscle fibers. Dr. Ghaheri describes it like delicately uncasing a sausage. The depth of the wound is still very shallow, maybe 1 mm or so, and in a baby the width is around 5 to 10 mm. Some people place sutures to close the wound, but a baby or child would need to be asleep for that step and, as we discussed earlier, the risk and cost of general anesthesia far outweigh the benefit of placing sutures.

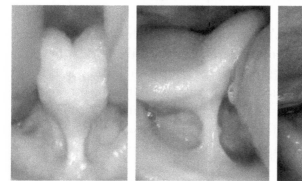
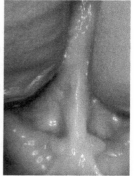

Previously clipped tongue-ties. Incomplete scissors releases often leave a thick band of restrictive tissue and little-to-no symptom relief. The anterior tongue-tie is iatrogenically made into a posterior tongue-tie. Releasing these fully results in symptom relief and improvement in nursing.[15]

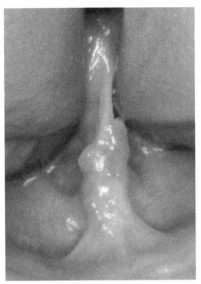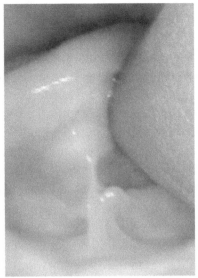

Examples of damaged salivary glands (left) and a cut into the body of the tongue (right). Incomplete scissors releases at the hospital left residual tension, continued symptoms, and caused iatrogenic damage by not cutting in the middle of the frenum. After a complete laser release, both mobility and symptoms improved.

Another method that is similar to scissors is cutting with a scalpel or sharp surgical knife. The blade has the same advantages and disadvantages as scissors, except if the child is awake and moving it can be more dangerous and can cut in undesirable locations, namely the lip or the large blood vessels in the floor of the mouth. These vessels are also at risk of being cut with scissors if the provider cannot see due to bleeding, is not using a light source (such as a headlamp), or magnification. The provider should not routinely use a hemostatic agent such as silver nitrate to stop bleeding. Silver nitrate is generally not necessary with a laser, and many practitioners have successfully performed scissors releases without using it as well. A surgeon can easily avoid the large vessels, thereby eliminating the need for silver nitrate. Silver nitrate is caustic and can leave a burn on the delicate tissue under the tongue, creating additional pain.

Cold gauze or gauze soaked in Afrin® (oxymetazoline) can also help stop bleeding, although firm pressure with gauze and allowing the baby to nurse right away will almost always stop the bleeding from a scissors or scalpel release. If significant bleeding is present, silver nitrate may be used, or additional emergent help should be sought to avoid further complications, either at the time of the procedure or in the postoperative period.

The next option is to use electrocautery, diathermy, or a Bovie (all basically the same thing) to burn the tissue so that it is obliterated. This method is typically the way it is performed if the child is asleep under general anesthesia, or if a non-laser surgeon performs it in the office. Many surgeons use cautery or Bovie to cut other tissues and get bleeding to stop when performing most surgeries in the operating room. The benefit of cautery is that it can provide a perfect view of the frenum and surgical area because there is minimal to no bleeding during cutting. The downside is that the child experiences more pain during and after the procedure because it burns and uses electricity. The depth of the energy and collateral damage that is created goes much deeper into the tissue than when other methods are used, and is therefore more painful because more nerves are involved. Compared to the laser, the Bovie can also result in slower wound healing, with increased scarring and a more significant inflammatory response. Another downside of cautery is that it can arc (depending on the type) and cause a burn on the lip that can leave a permanent scar. This happens if the Bovie touches any metal instrument while it is working.

The last and arguably the best option is to use a laser. Some might assert that using a laser is overkill, but they are likely not familiar with the way a laser performs surgically. Surgical use of a laser is not new, as the first CO_2 laser was invented in 1964 by Dr. Kumar Patel, and the first use of the CO_2 laser in oral surgery occurred in 1977. The laser is safer, gentler, more precise, and offers many advantages compared to the alternative methods described above. For these reasons, providers that perform these procedures on a regular basis should consider investing in a laser to provide these benefits to their patients and achieve consistently exceptional results from the surgery.

Proper use of a laser requires taking a laser safety course and implementing all laser safety protocols. The provider should be familiar with the laser's wavelength and properties, and he or she should take continuing–education courses to fully understand the parameters and best techniques in order to achieve the best results clinically. There is also a board certification available from the American Board of Laser Surgery that certifies medical doctors, dentists, and other healthcare professionals by written and oral examination. The process of certification helps providers understand and use lasers in a safe and effective manner.

There are two main types of surgical or dental lasers: contact and non-contact lasers. The first type, a contact laser, includes the diode laser which uses a quartz glass fiber that, after being initiated, uses laser energy to concentrate heat at the end of the tip, and the hot tip is touched to the tissue to perform a cut. The second type, a non-contact laser, includes erbium and CO_2 lasers which use an invisible beam in which the laser energy itself cuts the tissue without physically touching it with the handpiece. Both of these types of lasers work better than scissors, scalpel, or cautery because the surgeon can see the surgical field with little-to-no bleeding and consistently provide a precise cut.

The diode laser is less expensive and therefore more common than the other types of dental lasers. There are different brands of diode laser, but they all concentrate heat at the end of the glass fiber and require the provider to gently press on the tissue and use the heated fiber to cut the tongue, lip, or gums. The diode lasers must be "initiated" first, which is a process using a piece of dark paper, cork, or black ink on the tip to block the laser energy so it can reach operating temperature. The laser tip can get white hot, up to 900 to 1500 degrees Celsius![42,43] The heat causes the tissue to char and disappear, similar to the electrocautery, but the depth of the cut and resulting damage to underlying tissue is less than what occurs with cautery. The diode lasers typically take about a minute per site to work (so upper and lower frenum releases would take around 2 minutes). They are valuable tools but still require proper training to use effectively. As Dr. Ghaheri reminds practitioners in his lectures, just owning a laser does not make a surgeon competent. A good scissors release can result in a better outcome than a mediocre laser release.

The CO_2 and erbium classes are non-contact lasers. The provider hovers the tip of the laser over the tissue and the invisible laser energy goes into the tissue and heats up the water molecules in the tissue to 100 degrees Celsius, which is the boiling point of water. The water in the tissue located in the path of the beam turns to steam, taking the tissue with it, a process called vaporization. This process is very precise and removes tissue layers thinner than a human hair at a time. It creates less collateral damage to the underlying tissue than diode or cautery. The CO_2 laser produces less bleeding than the erbium class of lasers. This attribute is due to the wavelength used and additional properties that are beyond the scope of this book.

> *Owning a laser does not make a surgeon competent. A good scissors release can result in a better outcome than a mediocre laser release.*
> *– Bobby Ghaheri, MD*

Both types of dental lasers have been around for decades and have excellent safety records. They are used surgically at very low power, typically one to two watts, so there is no risk of cutting where they shouldn't. In fact, for a moving infant who is safely swaddled during the procedure, and for the patient, provider, and assistant who are wearing laser safety glasses, it is a much safer procedure than the scissors, scalpel or cautery methods. The laser only works when it is activated by a switch or foot pedal; otherwise, it cannot cut. And due to the low power settings, it also has to be in contact with the tissue (diode) for an extended period or aimed at the tissue (CO_2) for more than a few seconds to start cutting. If the patient moves, it is not a problem; nothing is cut unintentionally. The CO_2 laser is faster during the procedure because it cuts more efficiently;

it takes 5 to 10 seconds for the tongue and 10 to 20 seconds for the lip. That's a total of 15 to 30 seconds of treatment time compared with an average of two minutes when using most diodes. Two minutes of a baby crying versus 15 to 30 seconds is a big difference! If the provider has experience using the laser and knows how to operate it safely, it is both safe and effective at releasing tight frena with minimal bleeding and less pain than traditional methods. I noticed a much faster surgical time and decreased postoperative pain for the infants as reported by the mothers after switching from the diode to CO_2.

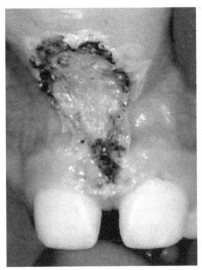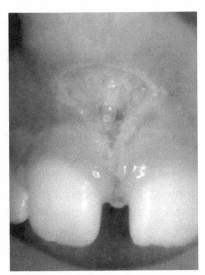

Laser wounds immediately after the procedure. Diode laser wound (left) and CO_2 laser wound (right).

Note: some of the photographs in this book show wounds that might look alarming to parents or non-surgeons. The wound itself is very superficial, with little to no bleeding, and oral tissues heal very rapidly and completely—usually with minimal scarring.

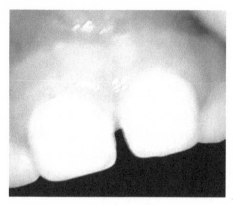

Both laser wounds heal nicely. Picture of the same diode wound completely healed 6 weeks later.

A distinction between frenotomy, frenectomy, and frenuloplasty should also be made at this point. A snip or clip with scissors or using a scalpel to make a small cut is considered a frenotomy. When scissors, cautery, or a laser removes or excises the frenum, this is more appropriately called a frenectomy because the tissue is physically removed by excision, cautery, ablation, or vaporization. Some may use the term "frenulectomy" to refer to the same thing as a frenectomy, but it is more of a tongue-twister and the term comes from referring to the "frenum" as a "frenulum." These terms are often used interchangeably, but sometimes a "frenulum" refers to a smaller "frenum." Finally, "frenuloplasty" refers to a procedure involving sutures in which multiple cuts are made, two triangular pieces are rotated to form a "Z" shape and then sutured in place. It can also be done by making a horizontal cut with scissors or a laser and suturing it vertically to close it. The frenuloplasty is a more complicated procedure and requires general anesthesia when performed on a baby or young child, so it is not recommended and is not typically necessary. It's not surprising that there is confusion regarding the names of the operations, given that there are four different terms in the literature describing very similar procedures!

Before the Procedure

Before the procedure begins, examination and history forms are completed (see Appendix for sample forms), and informed consent is obtained. Informed consent means there has been a discussion between the parents or patient and the provider about the procedure and all of the potential risks, benefits, and alternatives to treatment. Once all the information is presented, and the parents wish to proceed with surgery, the consent form is signed.

The most significant risk is mild-to-moderate bleeding at the surgical site. This risk is minimized by using a light source, such as a headlamp, and magnification so the surgical site is easily visualized. The risk is also decreased by the surgeon's skill and proficiency with the procedure. The wider the release and broader the diamond, the greater the chance of hitting the veins in the floor of the mouth, which can cause bleeding. In addition, the wider the diamond, the greater the risk of reattachment. For this reason, the diamond-shaped release should be kept as narrow as possible but still allow for full mobility of the tongue.

The diamond should be kept as narrow as possible but still allow for full mobility of the tongue.

After the procedure, there can be complications, such as reattachment. This phenomenon is discussed in detail in the next chapter, but all wounds contract during the healing process, and exercises or therapy must be done to prevent the upper and lower parts of the wound from sticking to each other as they heal. These exercises come with their own risks (e.g., an oral aversion in the child) if they are not performed gently enough. Although an aversion is rare, it can cause a baby to balk when anything such as a bottle, nipple, fingers, or pacifier is placed in his mouth. These risks are all uncommon, but precautions should be taken to avoid the risk of bleeding, reattachment, and oral aversion.

During the Procedure

For small babies and young children, it is often helpful to use special equipment (such as an infant swaddle for babies) and a second assistant to keep the patient still during the procedure. Laser safety goggles are placed on the patient, and are worn by the assistants and doctor as well. Specialized positioning boards and gel donuts for the baby's head can also help with positioning.

Topical numbing jelly containing a mix of lidocaine and prilocaine may lessen the baby's discomfort during the procedure, but also carries some risks. Some advocate not using a topical jelly, as studies have shown minimal to no benefit with regard to crying and appearance of pain.[44,45] The babies typically cry during the procedure with or without jelly, and a crying baby is a healthy baby. Either approach is appropriate, and should be determined by each provider on a case-by-case basis. Sucrose (sugar) water can also help lessen pain, and is given during a heel stick or circumcision, but is not typically used during frenectomy because breast milk seems to work just as well, and sucrose water caries other risks. [46,47] However, 20% benzocaine (Orajel™ and others) should not be used on children younger than 2 years old because of the potential for causing methemoglobinemia, a serious condition that can result in trouble breathing, pale, grey, or blue lips and skin, and rapid heart rate.[48] Other local anesthetics could potentially cause this reaction as well, although it is very rare. If any of those signs are noted after administering a local anesthetic, call emergency services immediately. Before and after intraoral photographs of the surgical areas help create a visual record of the procedure for the patient's chart.

When performing the procedure, it is typically best if the parents are not in the room. With the parents in the laser treatment room, there is a risk that they may receive eye damage from the laser. A few parents become so nervous that they require attention themselves, when the focus should be on the child. The provider needs to keep 100% of his or her attention on the child. Because the procedure is very short, the separation from the parents is only a few minutes long.

The only potentially serious complication, which rarely occurs (fewer than 1 in 100 procedures when using the laser), is moderate bleeding. This problem is easily managed by holding some gauze in place to make sure the wound clots, or by using the other methods discussed above. Bleeding could become severe if larger vessels are cut, so providers must be prepared and have a plan in the event that more brisk bleeding occurs. The other reason to have the mother out of the room is that ideally the baby will nurse immediately after the surgery. If the mother is watching the procedure, she will undoubtedly be more stressed, and her increased adrenaline and stress will shut off milk ejection, which means less milk will come out when the baby tries to nurse. The typical amount of time the infant is away from the mother is about three minutes, and as soon as the baby is returned, he or she usually has already stopped crying and tries to nurse within a few minutes. It is easier to have parents present for the tongue-tie release in toddlers and older children if they wish. Further information on releasing ties in children and adults is discussed in Chapter 14.

CHAPTER 8

After the Procedure

If I were to make a small cut on my hand, the wound would close and heal over in a couple of weeks. Likewise, if I make a specialized cut under the tongue or the upper lip with a laser (or a different method), it will heal back together if it is not kept separated. Babies heal very rapidly, and wounds contract naturally. Although everyone heals at a different rate, the tongue typically heals in around three weeks, and the lip usually heals in about two weeks when stretching exercises are performed. Healing continues underneath the area after this, but the wound is mostly gone and it can be difficult to tell exactly where it was after that amount of time. The goal is for the wound to heal open with the edges separated and the cut to close by secondary intention, meaning that it will fill in on its own and not be closed right after the surgery with sutures. The key is to have the wound heal lengthwise and the sides to heal in toward each other instead of the top of the diamond sticking back down and causing a shortening of the tongue. Autumn R. Henning, MS, CCC-SLP, COM likes to say, "We want the curtains to close; we don't want the window to shut." Maximum movement and function of the tongue is the goal.

There is no research on the most effective stretching and exercise protocol. Some people call it exercises or aftercare stretches, but they're all referring to the same thing, which is essentially a way to keep the areas separated to prevent healing back together, termed "reattachment." The consensus is to recommend performing stretches for enough time that the risk of healing back together is minimized while trying to prevent the child from developing an aversion to having the stretches performed and possibly even retaining an oral aversion. We always want to be respectful of the baby and try to keep the exercises as playful as possible. The exercises should be gentle but use sufficient pressure, about the same amount of pressure as using an ink stamp on a stamp pad. Get in and get out.

There are strong opinions regarding the length of time, movement, and the number of times a day the stretches are needed. While I don't want to presume that this way is the best or only way, what follows is the consensus for aftercare. Most practitioners suggest performing exercises ranging from 4 to 6 times a day for 2 to 6 weeks. One week of stretches (or no stretches at all) is, in my opinion, too short an amount of time and is more likely to result in reattachment. The exercises are less painful once the wound has closed, but they can still help maximize mobility of the tissue during postoperative weeks 3 to 6 if done playfully and gently.

We want the curtains to close; we don't want the window to shut. – Autumn Henning, MS, CCC-SLP, COM

The general motion is lifting the tongue and making sure there is tension on the wound and it appears as a skinny diamond—with the edges not sticking together. Using a camping headlamp or flashlight is very helpful, and I encourage parents to wear disposable medical gloves as well. If you can't see it, you can't stretch it. It is best not to rub vigorously directly on the wound, as you can cause more inflammation, leading to additional scar tissue formation. The tissue around the diamond turns a red and white splotchy color if this occurs (it is not infected, just inflamed). A gentle rolling-pin motion can be helpful on top of the wound, and it might be best after it has started healing to lengthen the wound as it tries to heal back together. Make funny noises or tickle the child's nose if they're a little older to avoid creating an aversion.

For a lip stretch, lift the lip up to the nostrils. Don't just roll the lip outward, but rather sink your fingers all the way into the fold under the lip (the vestibule) and lift it outward and up; the whole diamond-shaped wound should be visible. The same goes for the tongue. Come from behind and place 2 index fingers under the tongue and lift or push the tongue back and up at the top of the diamond. Your fingers should be at the apex or top of the diamond in the middle, not to the sides of the diamond. It should reveal the entire diamond shape and hold the stretch for around 10 seconds. A video of the stretching exercises we recommend is on our website at www.TongueTieAL.com.

The wound will usually turn a white or yellow color, which is just the way the fibrin that makes up a scab in the mouth appears when it is wet. This wound does not need antibiotics, and there are no reports of one getting infected. I've performed thousands of procedures and have never seen one get infected. It is still good practice, however, to wash your hands or wear medical gloves before doing the exercises. I personally think the parents find it easier and less slippery to stretch when wearing gloves, which can be purchased at most drugstores.

Reattachment can happen relatively quickly if a good stretch isn't performed or if the parent can't visualize the wound. For example, a baby is doing great after the release and the mother's symptoms are better, but all of a sudden (at 7 to 10 days after surgery) the baby's symptoms begin to reappear and/or nursing becomes difficult for mom again. It is possible that the tongue or lip is reattaching. It is more often the tongue that reattaches because it is more difficult to visualize and access. If the symptoms start to come back, or if you suspect it is healing back together, then return to the provider's office for a follow-up visit as soon as possible. We encourage all of our patients to return for a one-week follow-up to check on the healing and offer any advice we can. At this visit, if the lip or tongue wound looks like it is healing back together, we will do a deeper stretch of the area with a gentle push that takes just a second. Often patients report that the symptoms go away again after the deeper stretch, and the nursing is much better. We also show the parents how to do the exercises again and encourage them to keep doing them, possibly more often or with more pressure than they were before, to prevent reattachment. The majority of cases in which we have had to repeat the procedure due to reattachment and return of symptoms (which is around 1% in our office) involved patients who did not return for the one-week follow-up visit. We don't perform the procedure again with the laser unless it has been more than a month or two after the release and symptoms have come back again.

If the symptoms start to come back, or if you suspect it is healing back together, return to the provider's office for a follow-up visit.

Pain Management

After the frenectomy procedure, the tongue is typically more sore than the lip area, primarily because the tongue is moving more than the lip during nursing (or chewing and speaking for older children). I have undergone both the lip and tongue releases with the CO_2 laser, and I didn't even take any pain medication with the lip frenectomy. I used only numbing jelly on my lip, and the sensation during the procedure wasn't too bad. The only over-the-counter pain medication for babies under six months is Tylenol® (acetaminophen). The dose is weight-based, and the dosing should be given to you by the release provider. Ibuprofen (Motrin®) dosed by weight is the pain reliever of choice for babies over six months old. I think that the benefits of pain control for the infant far outweigh the potential risks. Babies generally don't require more than a couple of days of pain medicine, and if they are uncomfortable they are less likely to eat.

Typically, the laser energy will numb the area for about 3 to 4 hours because it removes the nerve endings from that area. The scissors release doesn't have this effect because it is simply cutting through the nerve endings, so it is typically more painful afterward. A study comparing the pain after a scissors release versus a laser release in older children and adults showed that less pain was reported by those who had the CO_2 laser frenectomy.[49]

Homeopathic remedies for babies and children are available that are beyond the scope of this book, but if you're interested in this option, information can be found online or from your provider. *Arnica montana* is one option that can help calm the baby, along with Rescue Remedy, but these should only be used under the supervision of your care provider or a naturopathic or homeopathic practitioner. Other great options include things such as holding the baby skin-to-skin, playing soothing music to relax the baby, nursing (carefully) in the bathtub with warm water, dimming the lights, and giving a gentle massage to the baby. Breast milk ice chips can also be used, which involves taking frozen breast milk and breaking off small pieces that the baby can suck on or eat to help cool the area. Care must be taken to ensure the baby doesn't have too large a piece, and ice made from water is not advised because it is not a good idea to give a baby water at an early age.

Ways to calm the baby after a release: pain medicine, skin-to-skin, soothing music, gentle massage, warm bath, and breast milk ice chips.

What to Expect

After the procedure, about half of the parents notice a deeper latch to the breast (or bottle) in the office, and the other half often notice a difference soon after. Sometimes it takes a few days to weeks for the baby to re-learn how to suck and overcome the muscle memory that has existed since before birth. Babies begin swallowing around 20 weeks in utero, so even if the baby is only a few days old, there may be muscle patterns or compensations that have taken place that must be retrained. Often parents will notice a decrease in pain, an increase in milk taken from the breast, an increase in supply (increased demand leads to increased supply), decreased fussiness, less gassiness, and a decrease in reflux or spitting up. Sometimes the parents may notice an increase in drooling or in spitting up for a time, but it normally resolves once sucking patterns have changed.

It is important to realize that these things may occur at different times for different babies. It can feel like a roller coaster, with ups and downs, emotionally and physically. The stretches can become cumbersome, and parents often report that the exercises are the hardest part of the whole process. One lactation consultant we work with says to expect one better feed per day; in other words, one good feed the first day, two good feeds the second day, and so on. Another says success is measured in weeks, not in days, so next week should be better than this week. Some people experience immediate relief, while others take longer, but if the mother keeps up with the aftercare exercises and follows up with her lactation consultant and any other needed referrals, it often gets significantly better by the third week. Again, if the symptoms get better and then come back around day 7 or 10, the tongue or lip could be reattached, so make a follow-up visit with your release provider. If the pain is worse on one side, or the latch is better on one side rather than the other, there may be an issue that requires assessment by a physical therapist, chiropractor, or craniosacral therapist for tight muscles or connective tissue (see Chapters 24 and 25).

CHAPTER 9

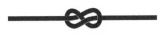

The Research

As we mentioned, there are more than 500 scientific studies involving tongue-ties. There also are more than 65,000 members of a social media group of moms with babies who have tongue-ties. Tongue-ties are clearly experiencing a resurgence of interest after decades of being left out of the medical and dental curriculum and, accordingly, clinical practice. This chapter examines some recent studies to determine if releasing the tongue is supported by evidence.

First, let's look at the different levels of evidence, some of which are of higher quality than others, with case studies being the lowest level of evidence above simply a doctor's opinion. Next are case-control studies followed by cohort studies. The gold-standard randomized controlled trials (taking subjects and splitting them into two groups randomly and then either treating or not treating) are one level up from the cohort study. Finally, a systematic review, which examines available studies and combines them to make one larger study sample on which to perform statistics is the highest level of evidence. To date, there are many case studies on tongue-ties, a few cohort studies, many randomized controlled trials, and just a few reviews of the available literature.

Most of the studies looked at procedures performed with scissors, and almost every study found that there is a benefit to releasing the tongue for nursing. Additionally, most of the studies report that it is a low-risk procedure with excellent benefits, and that more research on this topic is needed. There are some great articles from high-quality, reputable, peer-reviewed journals (such as *Pediatrics*) that should gain the respect and attention of the healthcare providers who are joining us in reading this book. Please read this section with an open mind, and leave the baggage from previous teachers and textbooks at the door for just a moment.

The availability of instant feedback from a massive audience of peers is the new paradigm of the Information Age, and it is not going away anytime soon. Now, with Google and Facebook, parents can instantly tell 1,000 of their friends not to use your office. So let's use the research and current clinical knowledge to make helpful recommendations, reassure the patients struggling with tongue-ties, and be compassionate about their concerns. In the process, you will protect your practice and reputation from online scrutiny while benefiting families.

So what's the connection between a simple tongue-tie and difficulty nursing? A restricted tongue in a baby leads to a shallow or poor latch due to the tongue not being able to elevate normally. Many times people think that if the baby can stick the tongue out, then there's not a tongue-tie. Often the babies are quickly evaluated in the mother's arms or while still in the car seat—neither place allows for a full exam. The act of protrusion or sticking out the tongue isn't the key, but rather lifting the tongue or elevation is the key to nursing (as well as speech and solid feeding, as we'll see later).

Geddes et al. (2008)

A study by Geddes et al. (2008) published in the journal *Pediatrics* showed with ultrasound imaging that babies use their tongues in an up-and-down motion, which creates a vacuum that causes the milk to come out of the breast.[12] This is in contrast to the previously held belief that the tongue compresses and massages the nipple to get the milk out.[50] When we evaluate tongue-tied babies, they often have sucking blisters or calluses on the lips because they are overusing their lip and cheek muscles and trying to get milk out like a straw. Their cheeks pull in to create the vacuum instead of their tongue forming the negative pressure by rising and falling normally. This action creates an excessive force on the nipple and leads to nipple distortion (flattened or lipstick-shaped nipples), nipple damage, and cessation of breastfeeding. This study showed the importance of the middle portion of the baby's tongue to lift up to nurse correctly. In the study, after the tongue-tied babies had their tongues released, they nursed better, got more milk, and the mothers reported less pain. The authors reported that the tight frenum leads to an ineffective seal. The pinching and pain for the mothers resolved after the frenotomy (scissors release) in 95% of mothers. Before the release, during nursing the babies were transferring an average of 5.6 mL of milk per minute. After the release, they transferred an average of 10.5 mL of milk per minute. The tongue-tied babies received around half as much milk per suck as non-tongue-tied babies and therefore would get tired or nurse for extended periods of time. The mothers also experienced an increase in their milk supply because the babies were taking more milk (increased demand leads to increased supply). The 24-hour milk production of six mothers measured increased after the release—an average of 160 g in just seven days. This study, which was published in a highly reputable journal, adds to the evidence base and shows a real, measurable benefit to releasing the tongue in addition to helping us understand how babies extract milk. Knowing why the procedure helps the baby nurse better is critical to understanding the proper examination process and how the release works to improve nursing. In addition, Elad (2014) confirmed the findings of the study using ultrasound imaging and 3D modeling.[51]

The tongue-tied babies received around half as much milk per suck as non-tongue-tied babies.

They determined that infants generate negative pressure of –20 to –40 mmHg for milk extraction instead of chewing on the nipple.

Hogan et al. (2005)

An article from 2005 by Hogan showed that out of all of the babies born in a particular hospital (1866 births) who were assessed, 201 (10.7%) had a tongue-tie (anterior or visible tongue-tie only).[16] They decided to test to see if releasing the tongue made a difference. They randomized 57 of the babies and gave half of them lactation support (control group) and half of them a tongue-tie release with scissors. The average age at release was three weeks old. They saw 96% improvement in the group that had the tongue-tie released, whereas the control group had only a 3% improvement from lactation support alone. Next, they offered the control group the release at 48 hr, and 96% of those babies also improved. Overall, 54 of 57 babies improved from the tongue-tie release, which means 95% of babies saw an improvement. The authors stated that "there is no need to release all tongue-ties at birth, but awareness of the relationship of tongue-ties with feeding problems will allow release in symptomatic babies to be performed without delay." This statement points out the fact that many babies appear tied, but in fact feed adequately (at least in the beginning). But mothers should nonetheless be made aware of the presence of a tie so if they have issues in the future, such as poor latch, painful nursing, or supply issues, they can seek help and not feel confused. Mothers often blame themselves if their babies can't feed well, thinking they just have flat nipples or insufficient glandular tissue, when in reality it is an anatomic problem with the baby.

Conversely, providers sometimes blame the baby and say, "He's just a lazy nurser," or that his mouth is just "too small," neither of which makes sense from a survival-evolutionary standpoint. Babies need and want to eat, instinctively. On the other hand, if there are symptoms present, then these tongue-ties should be released as soon as possible to give the mother-baby dyad the best chance of a great nursing relationship. The article goes on to say that "what was important was not the length of the tongue-tie, but the symptoms it was causing." If a baby has a maxillary frenum or lingual frenum (as almost all do), but there are no issues, then no procedure is necessary. They are both normal anatomical findings when they are elastic and not overly tight or thick. However, if there is a functional problem, it is best to fix it sooner rather than later for the sake of the mother and the baby (and don't forget poor dad, too!). A breastfeeding screening questionnaire is helpful for a pediatrician or OB/GYN to use at the one-week postpartum visit or subsequent visits to determine if any nursing issues are present (a sample infant questionnaire is included in the Appendix).

"There is no need to release all tongue-ties at birth, but awareness of the relationship of tongue-ties with feeding problems will allow release in symptomatic babies to be performed without delay."[16]

The Hogan article indicates that, although many of the doctors in their hospital agreed with the statement that "tongue-ties do not cause problems with feeding," none of the doctors' interventions, nor those of the lactation consultants (changing the positioning or hold), made the baby nurse better. However, by the end of the study, it was concluded that "feeding was improved by the simple, safe procedure of removing the physical problem which was preventing it—the tongue-tie." In case this isn't enough evidence to convince you, I've included a few more randomized controlled trials below.

Berry, Griffiths, and Westcott (2012)

Berry, Griffiths, and Westcott published their double-blind, randomized controlled trial of tongue-tie and its effect on breastfeeding in the journal *Breastfeeding Medicine*.[11] They took 57 babies younger than four months old and assessed their feeding capabilities for two minutes. They assessed LATCH scores and maternal pain scores on a scale from 1 to 10. Then they either performed the release with scissors, or they pretended to do it (a "sham" procedure) as a control group, and then assessed the same scores immediately. They told the mothers not to look into the baby's mouth until after they had fed again. They then offered the sham control group the release the same day because it is unethical to withhold treatment from a baby when the procedure has repeatedly demonstrated that it makes a significant difference. Seventy-eight percent of the treatment group mothers reported immediate improvement following the tongue-tie release. Interestingly, 47% of the sham group saw improvement (initially) as well, so there was a placebo effect, but the statistical difference between the two groups demonstrating the effectiveness of the intervention was still significant at p<0.02. Therefore, the placebo effect was not the reason for the difference the mothers experienced. Ninety percent of the babies who were released saw improvement at day one, and by three months 92% had improvement, so it was sustained. None of the mothers reported worse feeding, and all of the mothers said they would do the procedure again. The article states that "there is a real, immediate improvement in breastfeeding, detectable by the mother, which is sustained and *does not* appear to be due to a placebo effect" (emphasis added). The authors also stated that it is best if babies can be identified and treated for

"A real, immediate improvement in breastfeeding, detectable by the mother, which is sustained and does not appear to be due to a placebo effect"[11]

tongue-tie by two weeks of age. The younger the baby, the better they do at re-learning and overcoming compensations present since before birth.

Buryk, Bloom, and Shope (2011)

Here is one final randomized controlled trial that was published in the journal *Pediatrics* in 2011 and conducted by Buryk, Bloom, and Shope.[10] This was a blinded randomized controlled trial with 30 babies in the release group and 28 in the sham control group. Researchers used reliable and validated tools for measuring pain and breastfeeding scores, including the Hazelbaker Assessment Tool for Lingual Frenulum Function (HATLFF), which grades on appearance and function; the Short-Form McGill Pain Questionnaire (SF-MPQ) for assessing nipple pain; and an Infant Breastfeeding Assessment Tool (IBFAT). All of these assessments have been studied previously and shown to be valid and reliable tools. They found that the frenotomy group had significantly decreased pain (p<.001) compared to the sham group. The IBFAT showed that the frenotomy group had significantly fewer breastfeeding problems and significantly higher maternal satisfaction with breastfeeding (p=.029). All but one parent in the sham group asked to have the frenotomy at or before the two-week follow-up, so the researchers couldn't continue studying differences between the two groups. The article stated that "when frenotomy is performed for clinically significant ankyloglossia, there is a clear and immediate improvement in reported maternal nipple pain and infant breastfeeding scores." Furthermore, they "found the procedure to be rapid, simple, and without complications," and suggested that the optimal timing of frenotomy occurs sometime between two and six days after birth. Typically, the earlier the release is performed, the better and faster the baby will improve because he or she is not fighting muscle patterns and compensations that have been established for weeks and months. Finally, they discussed that "maternal nipple pain and poor infant latch are common reasons for early discontinuation of breastfeeding. There is evidence that ankyloglossia causes both poor latch and nipple pain compared with infants without ankyloglossia. Studies of frenotomy to relieve neonatal ankyloglossia have consistently shown a benefit." This statement is undoubtedly true because if the mothers have 10/10 pain every time the baby tries to eat, they are not going to continue nursing for 6 weeks, let alone the recommended 6 months or more.

> *"A clear and immediate improvement in reported maternal nipple pain and infant breastfeeding scores."[10]*

Many mothers report to us that they would rather endure unmedicated labor again than nurse the baby because the nursing pain is, in fact, worse than labor. If the baby can't latch well and is choking on milk, having reflux issues experiencing poor weight gain, not transferring milk, and seemingly always hungry, mom is going to give up and switch to formula and a bottle (although there are still tongue-tie issues with bottle-feeding). Many mothers tell us at the initial consult, "You are our last hope." The mothers plan to stop nursing if the pain and baby's nursing issues are not resolved because they are at their wit's end. Thankfully, almost all the mothers who have told us they are "about to give up" saw a benefit and were helped by the procedure enough to save the breastfeeding relationship. Breastfeeding exclusively for 6 months is promoted by the American Academy of Pediatrics (AAP) and other organizations,[8] and it is important to realize that if we're going to push this goal, we have to give the mothers the support they need and the tools they need to achieve the goal.

Posterior Ties

The first report of a posterior tongue-tie was from Betty Coryllos and Cathy Watson-Genna in 2004, [24] so the concept of the "posterior" tongue-tie is relatively new, medically speaking. The idea makes a lot of sense because for years people have known that there are some babies with tongue-tie symptoms but no distinguishing visible flag of a tie.

Chu and Bloom (2009)

For those who question the existence of posterior tongue-tie, here's a case-report from Chu and Bloom in 2009.[52] This article described a "rare entity" of a posterior tongue-tie. But was it rare, or just not diagnosed properly? The authors stated that the frenum was hidden by a "mucosal curtain," meaning it couldn't be seen without pulling back on the tissue, and then it popped up. They put the four-week-old baby to sleep (not ideal, as we now know) and used a hemostat to clamp the frenum, cut twice, achieved a "diamond" shape, and put in 4 sutures. They noted the mother had immediate relief of nursing pain and an improved latch. They called it a "safe, quick, and effective treatment that can provide immediate symptom relief, promote breastfeeding, and enhance infant-mother bonding experience." This study was published in the *International Journal of Pediatric Otorhinolaryngology* and helps to counteract the claims of those who deny the existence of the posterior tongue-tie. We see this scenario repeated multiple times daily at our office, where we release a posterior tongue-tie and the mother's and baby's symptoms improve significantly. Releasing a posterior tongue-tie can work wonders for families and is an effective treatment if the practitioner knows how to diagnose and release it properly. When providers merely clip the anterior portion of the tongue, they can actually turn the anterior tie into a posterior tie, as seen earlier. As a result, mom still has symptoms and the baby still won't latch well. If the posterior section is adequately released, the latch almost always improves, and the mother experiences less pain and fewer symptoms.

"A safe, quick, and effective treatment that can provide immediate symptom relief, promote breastfeeding, and enhance infant-mother bonding experience."[52]

O'Callahan, Macary and Clementine (2013)

A study by O'Callahan, Macary and Clementine (2013) showed the benefits of releasing the tongue-tie and lip-tie in 299 infants. [13] Most of the babies in the study (85%) referred for release by Dr. O'Callahan, a pediatrician, had a posterior tongue-tie. Latching issues and nipple pain significantly improved after the procedure (scissors release, $p<.001$). He used proper technique with scissors and reported a flat, diamond shape to the wound, and recommended stretching exercises for five days. It is best to stretch for longer, at least two weeks, but this is one of the only studies available that mentions stretching exercises at all. Ninety-four percent of mothers reported that there were no complications or adverse side effects, and 93% of those surveyed responded that the procedure was worth the physical and emotional discomfort to both themselves and the infants. Researchers mentioned that latching and pain issues often resolved around one week post-frenotomy and sometimes longer, depending on the baby. They also reported that the babies with a posterior tongue-tie were more likely to have a lip-tie than the babies with a classic anterior tongue-tie. In our office, our experience echoes these results—that almost all babies with a posterior tongue-tie have a lip-tie as well.

Ghaheri et al. (2017)

Another article that discusses releasing a posterior tongue-tie and the benefit to nursing is "Breastfeeding Improvement Following Tongue-Tie and Lip-Tie Release: A Prospective Cohort Study"[14] by Ghaheri et al. (2017). This study was helpful to the current literature regarding tongue-tie because it specifically addresses posterior tongue-ties, lip-ties, and reflux in infants, and was one of the only studies that utilized a dental laser for the release. Dr. Ghaheri is an ENT who is well known in tongue-tie professional circles, and has helped countless babies with nursing issues. This study looked at factors such as milk transfer rate, maternal self-confidence, pain scores, and reduction in infant reflux symptoms. They found that the babies with a posterior tongue-tie improved after release, much like anterior tongue-tie (to-the-tip or almost-to-the-tip) babies did following release. On all of the validated scores (meaning they have been shown to be real and measurable in other studies), the babies improved significantly—their reflux improved from 16.5 to 13.2 to 11.6, indicating the reflux symptoms (including spitting up) decreased or went away. The maternal self-confidence scores improved after the release greater than the pivotal score of 50. If the score is below 50, the mothers are likely to stop nursing, whereas above 50 they will likely continue nursing. The scores went from 43.9 before the surgery to a 56.5 one month later, which means that before the procedure these moms were likely to stop nursing and give up, but afterward they felt they could continue breastfeeding.

We hear weekly in the office that "I've been to two other providers who say there's no problem, but I can't take the pain anymore, and I'm about to give up." According to the Ghaheri et al. study, the frenectomy helps these moms feel like they can keep going and gives them hope of pain and symptom relief. The pain for mothers in this study decreased from an average of 4.6/10 before surgery to 2.2/10 at one week and barely any pain with an average of 1.5/10 at one month. Dr. Ghaheri and his team treated lip-ties if indicated and posterior tongue-ties, and used a dental laser. This article is a great addition to the literature because he used the currently preferred method by experts worldwide and achieved a full release to provide relief for these moms and babies who were struggling. Many of the other articles available in the literature utilized the simple "snip" or "clip," as has been performed for centuries. Dr. Ghaheri, however, provided a more contemporary full release of the connective tissue and mucosa back to the genioglossus muscle, leaving a diamond-shaped wound and

Mothers often report, "I can't take the pain anymore, and I'm about to give up."

95

removing the entire frenum, both anterior and posterior portions. He also recommended stretching exercises 4 to 6 times a day for several weeks.

Pransky, Lago, and Hong (2015)

A retrospective study by Pransky, Lago, and Hong (2015) was conducted while they were working in an ENT specialty clinic. They reported seeing a large number of posterior tongue-tie and hypothesized that the true incidence rate of tongue-tie (including posterior) is likely higher than what is currently reported.[26] This article is helpful because it specifies how many infants had anterior ties, posterior ties, and the combination of lip-tie associated with each variant or alone. In their results, 78% of the mothers saw an improvement in breastfeeding, with 61% saying it was significant. Of note, 91% of patients with posterior tongue-tie (120 babies) also saw improvement. Considering babies with upper lip-tie only, 79% improved, and babies with both anterior tongue-tie and lip-tie saw 91% improvement. Babies with posterior tongue-tie and lip-tie saw 85% improvement. They also noted that 21% of babies referred to them had no oral cavity anomalies, which indicated that there are "multiple reasons why a newborn may have breastfeeding difficulties."

Ghaheri, Cole, and Mace (2018)

The most recently published study (at the time of writing) is from Ghaheri, Cole, and Mace (2018), which describes how babies with prior incomplete releases and persistent breastfeeding issues see benefit from a complete laser release.[15] In the three measures, the same used in the 2017 article described earlier—the breastfeeding self-efficacy score, the GERD questionnaire, and a visual analog scale of pain during breastfeeding—all participants saw improvement at one week and one month postoperatively. The breastfeeding score went from 45.1 at baseline to 52.1 at one week and 56.9 at one month, indicating the mothers felt they could continue nursing successfully. Again, scores below 50 are associated with breastfeeding cessation. The GERD symptoms decreased from 15.7 to 11.9 at one week and 10.4 at one month. The mother's pain decreased from an initial mean of 4.8/10 to 2.2 at one week, and 1.6 at one month, indicating a better latch and much less pain. In this article, the researchers also describe the technique we advocate: removing the midline tissue in the residual frenum and then extending a "central window" bilaterally with a "diamond-shaped incision that is flush with the adjacent floor of the mouth tissue." As stated previously, the shape results naturally from an incision through a triangular frenum and is indicative of a complete release. Importantly, they note that "children who have not improved following a previous frenotomy may have further restriction under the tongue that still needs attention." This statement could also be said of older children and adults. Incomplete releases are, unfortunately, commonplace, and this study adds to the evidence base that releasing these already clipped frenums in those with continuing symptoms does, in fact, improve measurable outcomes and breastfeeding longevity.

> *"Children who have not improved following a previous frenotomy may have further restriction under the tongue that still needs attention."*[15]

As discussed in the 2017 study led by Ghaheri, reflux is a common problem seen in infants that is often treated with histamine (H_2) blockers such as Zantac® (ranitidine) or a proton pump inhibitor (PPI) such as Prilosec, Prevacid®, or Nexium® (esomeprazole). None of the PPIs are FDA-approved for use in infants. In many cases, babies with tongue-ties display signs of reflux and are put on a PPI medication, gripe water, or simethicone instead of investigating the real cause of the reflux. When one of our daughters was spitting up considerable amounts of milk from breast or bottle, and we had mountains of laundry and tried everything to help her keep milk down, my wife and I were told that the problem was purely "cosmetic." Even after Zantac®, gripe water, simethicone, and never laying her flat (even while sleeping), she still suffered, and it didn't seem to make a difference. She choked on milk, turned blue, and it was frightening for us as first-time parents.

Siegel (2016)

For these infants with breastfeeding and bottle-feeding issues and a tongue-tie, one of the main indicators of a potential problem is a clicking or smacking noise heard while they eat due to an inadequate seal on the breast or bottle. However, a baby can also be swallowing air without the telltale clicking or smacking noise. In many cases, simply switching to a bottle and formula does NOT solve the problems experienced by families with tongue-tied babies. Siegel (2016) published an article titled "Aerophagia Induced Reflux in Breastfeeding Infants with Ankyloglossia and Shortened Maxillary Labial Frenulum (Tongue- and Lip-Tie),"[23] which discusses the phenomenon of aerophagia (eating air) that is seen after feeding and can be diagnosed by auscultation during feeding, colic-like symptoms after feeding, and gastric distention immediately after a feed (it can be seen on x-ray with an enlarged gastric bubble). Aerophagia and the clicking noises often disappear after a frenectomy, sometimes right away and in some cases it takes a few weeks. Sometimes just releasing the tongue will improve the situation, but often the tongue-tie and lip-tie (if present) need to be removed to see full improvement. In Dr. Siegel's practice, out of 1,000 infants treated with reflux symptoms, 526 (52.6%) saw improvement in their reflux symptoms and were able to wean off or decrease their medication; 191 (or 19.1%) of the babies improved in irritability, but still needed medication. And 283 (or 28.3%) did not improve, so there was likely another cause of their reflux. Does every child on Zantac® or Nexium® have a tongue-tie? Probably not, but it should be the first thing on the differential diagnosis list for reflux, especially in the presence of other tongue-tie symptoms and nursing difficulties. Primary care providers should do a proper assessment and history for tongue-tie if there are signs such as clicking noises, poor latch, poor seal, spitting up often, fussiness after eating, or excessive gas, all of which are very common issues in infants that parents are often told are "normal."

Finally, there are no randomized controlled trials on only releasing lip-ties and its effect on breastfeeding as there are for tongue-ties. In the Pransky article, there was a subset of 14 babies who underwent lip-tie release only and 78% saw improvement.[26] In our office, we have seen firsthand how lip-ties can affect nursing, and many other practitioners have seen this as well. The variability in the morphology and characteristics of the lip-tie and the complex interplay between tongue and lips and the concomitant tongue-tie with most lip-ties precludes the ability to tease out the lip-tie variable for a study on solely lip-ties. They are, however, described in the literature relating specifically to breastfeeding in several articles beginning around 1999.[19] Kotlow (2004) describes how a tight maxillary frenum can interfere with latching and nursing when it is restrictive,[17] Kotlow (2010) also describes how a tight maxillary frenum or lip-tie could contribute to decay on the maxillary anterior teeth because of difficulty brushing and retaining milk in the pocket next to the front teeth.[53]

As previously stated, we see babies who have only had a tongue-tie release and are still having nursing difficulties. When we subsequently release the lip-tie, they have a resolution of nursing symptoms and a deeper latch with a better seal, less clicking, less reflux and spitting up, and they transfer more efficiently. Keep an eye on the lip-tie if there are lingering nursing difficulties after a tongue-tie release, and treat if indicated. It may just be the missing piece of the puzzle.

Section 2: Feeding

"There is no love sincerer than the love of food."
— *George Bernard Shaw*

Food. There are lots of images, emotions, and memories that come to mind when someone even mentions food. Thanksgiving turkey. Christmas ham. New Year's Day pork, cabbage, and black eyed peas. Nearly every holiday and family event is centered around food and mealtimes. From the very beginning until the bitter end, it is our best friend, and our worst enemy. We like certain foods and can't stand others. We often take feeding and food for granted. Eat too much or too little and you're going to have problems.

With children, struggles with food can become a life-altering issue. When a child refuses to eat or is stubborn with food, we often blame the child or ourselves. As a parent holding a newborn baby, your number-one priority in life is keeping them healthy and safe. But what if keeping them healthy is a constant struggle because they aren't able to eat? For many babies, toddlers, and adolescents struggling with feeding, an underlying issue such as a tongue-tie may be to blame. Feeding progress can be made swiftly with a release of the tongue-tie and the help of feeding therapists, and the parent and child can get back to enjoying food and mealtimes instead of dreading them.

This section discusses in detail liquid feeding, purees, and solids, as well as what evaluation and treatment looks like from the point of view of a therapist and a provider. Finally, we conclude with the research chapter and discuss some cases reported in the literature (which are from our office) and how a tongue-tie impacted those children.

CHAPTER 10

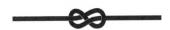

A Brief Overview of Feeding

Megan Musso, MA, CCC-SLP

Feeding is one of the most complex tasks our body undertakes. There are 6 cranial nerves and 26 muscles involved in feeding, and it takes all the systems of the body to process and use the food we eat. There are 8 muscle pairs directly connected to or within the tongue itself involved in feeding. As you can imagine, for a tongue-tied baby who may have impaired swallowing or tongue movement, this process can be especially difficult.

The act of swallowing is a coordinated dance between several muscles and reflexes, and takes place across four phases. In a mature swallow pattern, during the oral prep phase with the lips closed, the tongue, cheeks, and jaw begin to chew in a rotary (circular) fashion to make a food bolus. With liquids, the bolus is held on top of the tongue while it is pressed against the hard palate so it doesn't spill into the cheeks. The soft palate moves down against the tongue to close off the throat so none of the food is swallowed prematurely. Next, during the oral phase of about 1 to 1.5 seconds, the tongue elevates from front to back in a wavelike motion to propel the food toward the throat. Once the food is in the back of the mouth, it triggers a swallow reflex. During the pharyngeal phase of about 1 second, the muscles in the soft palate elevate to close off the nose, and the pharynx or throat area accepts the food bolus while the tongue retracts and creates pressure to force the food down.

Simultaneously, the hyoid bone in the neck lifts up to move the voice box out of the way and the epiglottis closes off the trachea so food doesn't enter the airway. This airway protection occurs at three levels: at the vocal folds, false vocal folds, and the base of the epiglottis. The food travels down the esophagus for about 8 to 20 seconds, as the muscles relax and contract like a wave (known as peristalsis) to move the food into the stomach. Valves called the upper esophageal sphincter and lower esophageal sphincter allow food to enter the esophagus and leave the esophagus for the stomach.

As you can see, the act of feeding is complex and requires the timely coordination of a great number of muscles and reflexes to work efficiently and safely. Because this process begins with the tongue, you can imagine the impact that tongue-tie can have on feeding, whether it be liquids or solids. This mature swallow pattern is not used at birth; babies are born with more simple reflexes, and these skills are learned over time through appropriate feeding experiences. Between birth and three years of age, babies to toddlers must learn how to use their oral structures in new and diverse ways to reach the goal of a mature chew/swallow pattern. A hiccup at any one of these milestones can greatly impact development of the oral musculature as well as patterns required for efficient and safe feeding.

Many great resources are available for lactation consultants, speech-pathologists, occupational therapists, pediatricians, parents, and other feeding therapists that do an amazing job of outlining typical feeding development and how to promote acquisition of appropriate skills. If I were to attempt to outline every muscle, reflex, movement pattern, and progression of feeding, you would probably put this book down before you reached the good stuff, so I encourage you to seek out the following resources if you are a professional or parent interested in this area:

» *Nobody Ever Told Me (or My Mother) That!*—Diane Bahr, MS, CCC-SLP, CIMI
» *Feed Your Baby and Toddler Right: Early Eating and Drinking Skills Encourage the Best Development*—Diane Bahr, MS, CCC-SLP, CIMI
» *Raising a Healthy Happy Eater: A Stage-by-Stage Guide to Setting Your Child on the Path to Adventurous Eating*—Melanie Potock, MA, CCC-SLP, & Nimali Fernando, MD, MPH
» *Baby Self-Feeding: Solutions for Introducing Purees and Solids to Create Lifelong, Healthy Eating Habits*—Melanie Potock, MA, CCC-SLP, & Nancy Ripton
» *Pre-Feeding Skills: A Comprehensive Resource for Mealtime Development*—Suzanne Evans Morris, PhD, CCC-SLP, & Marsha Dunn Klein, M. ED., OTR/L
» *Supporting Sucking Skills in Breastfeeding Infants*—Catherine Watson-Genna, BS, IBCLC
» Feeding Matters Online Resource: http://www.feedingmatters.org

Feeding development, as described by Dana Hearnsberger, a speech-language pathologist and feeding expert, begins in the center of the mouth. Using the proximal-distal (inside → outside) theory, her diagrams best explain how the tongue evolves in terms of movement and integration as we progress from liquid foods such as milk or formula to regular table foods.

Does feeding follow a predictable progression of physical skill development like other motor skills? YES!
Feeding begins in the center of the mouth. Oral motor skill development for feeding moves out proximodistally from midline tongue and palate to lateral tongue then ultimately to gums-teeth.

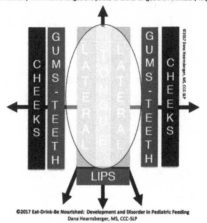

©2017 Eat-Drink-Be Nourished: Development and Disorder in Pediatric Feeding
Dana Hearnsberger, MS, CCC-SLP

Reprinted with permission.[54]

At birth, a suckle pattern (50% anterior and 50% posterior movement) is used in which the tongue rests over the lower gum and grooves or cups the nipple, pulling it deeply to the junction of the hard and soft palate, while the posterior third of the tongue moves downward to create negative pressure. The rolling or wave-like motion of the tongue, along with the generated negative pressure, extracts the milk. Sucking pads (developed during the last month of pregnancy) are fat pads located on the inside of both cheeks. These keep the tongue stable at the midline, preventing liquid from entering the cheeks, and limit the oral space to make it easier to generate the necessary negative pressure to extract milk. Dr. Hazelbaker describes this pattern as akin to an octopus' arm moving freely and untethered in a wavelike motion from the center of its body to the very tip of the arm.[55] If there is any restriction or interruption in movement, the octopus would not be able to function and navigate the sea as it does.

Around 3 to 4 months of age, this suckle reflex begins to diminish and a different pattern emerges—the suck. During this time, a baby's mouth is changing: suck pads are getting smaller as the cheek muscles strengthen, and the oral cavity in general is growing in space. These changes lead to the tongue having more freedom to move with increased responsibilities. Before, when the oral cavity was much smaller, the front-to-back movement coupled with the downward motion of the posterior third of the tongue was enough to create a vacuum to extract milk; now the process becomes more complicated. A suck pattern emerges as the lateral margins and anterior third of the tongue begin to elevate toward the palate to seal and compress the nipple. The tongue, jaw, and lips begin to move independently of one another and must coordinate their movements precisely to facilitate the positive and negative pressure now required to extract milk. Positive pressure is established as the tongue tip and margins elevate to the palate with the jaw elevated and lips sealed around the nipple. Negative pressure required to extract the milk is established as the jaw depresses, cheeks contract, soft palate elevates, and tongue depresses from the hard palate. As you can see, there are a lot of muscles and movements to be coordinated in the complicated dance of breastfeeding or bottle-feeding.

Arguably one of the most important changes for feeding development between 4 and 6 months of age is the increasing strength in oral structures, as well as differentiation (independent movement) of these structures. During this period of growth, baby learns to move the tongue while keeping the jaw, cheeks, and lips stable. This skill is critical for future feeding and speech success. Teeth may begin to emerge during this period, and babies have increased oral experiences and may be ready for purees, soft cookies, and the introduction of open cup drinking (with assistance).

Babies at 6 to 12 months of age are exposed to new adventures, including purees, straw/open cup drinking, and solids. The gag reflex has moved to the posterior third of the tongue, and the transverse tongue reflex (sideways tongue movement toward a stimulus) begins to develop. The transverse tongue reflex is activated with touch to the sides of the tongue or gums. This reflex is critical later on for moving food to and from the gum/teeth surfaces during chewing. A suck or suckle pattern is used for purees and liquids initially with some munching (up and down movement of jaw). Diagonal chewing is observed when foods are placed laterally in the mouth, such as meltables or soft solids.

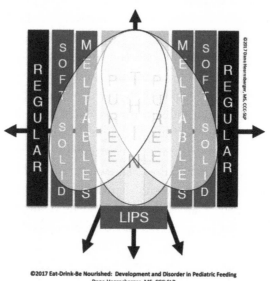

©2017 Eat-Drink-Be Nourished: Development and Disorder in Pediatric Feeding
Dana Hearnsberger, MS, CCC-SLP

Reprinted with permission.[54]

With exposure over time to new consistencies and foods, the primitive suck and suckle patterns, transverse tongue reflex, and munching pattern diminish, with a more mature swallow pattern evolving around 12 to 18 months of age. A mature swallow pattern is initiated with the tongue tip to the alveolar ridge (the bumps behind the front teeth). At this time, toddlers should be biting through soft cookies with ease, using coordinated diagonal rotary chewing (jaw is moving diagonally, to the side and back to center) and lateralizing the tongue with increased precision. By 2 years of age, a child should start using a mature chew pattern, known as rotary (circular) chewing. This chew pattern is what adults use (or should use) and occurs when the jaw moves in a circle to grind the food with the tongue constantly placing food back on the teeth surfaces for chewing.

Babies may master or develop these skills a little bit earlier or later than mentioned above; however, feeding development (like other developmental skills) occurs on a continuum. If a child skips one of these feeding milestones, it will likely adversely affect future development of oral structures and/or patterns.

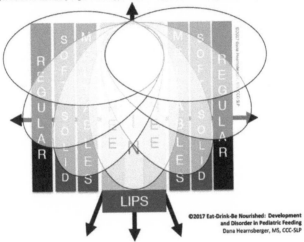

PROGRESSION OF FOOD TEXTURE + ORAL MOTOR SKILLS

As a child's progression of oral motor skills for lateralization and early chewing (munching) develops, child begins transition from purees and meltables to foods with more texture. As chewing skills progress from munching (up-down jaw pattern) to more advanced rotary-diagonal chewing pattern, child begins transition to regular texture foods.

©2017 Eat-Drink-Be Nourished: Development and Disorder in Pediatric Feeding
Dana Hearnsberger, MS, CCC-SLP

Reprinted with permission.[54]

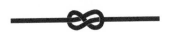

CHAPTER 11

Liquid Feeding
(Bottles, Cups, and Straws)
Megan Musso, MA, CCC–SLP

We hear a lot about how ties can impact nursing, but what about bottle-feeding? Bottle-feeding requires the use of many of the same muscles, but with a different motor pattern. As previously discussed, seal, oral control, and suck-swallow-breathe are all required for successful bottle-feeding as well as nursing. In contrast to breastfeeding, bottle-feeding babies must use more cheek and lip movement. Fewer sucking movements are seen with shorter pauses in between suck bursts. Breastfeeding babies must create a vacuum to express the milk from the breast in addition to compressing the nipple, whereas bottle-feeding babies must simply compress the nipple to receive milk.

Sometimes bottle-feeding is easier than breastfeeding for tied babies. This is because the bottle nipple is already reaching the back of the mouth, and the baby does not need to lift and lower the back of the tongue to pull the nipple in, as with breastfeeding. Additionally, the baby does not have to "wait and work" to get the milk, as bottles flow freely in contrast to a milk letdown in breastfeeding. However, for some tied babies, breastfeeding is the easier option. In the case of oversupply/strong letdown, the baby is able to more passively drink from the breast; therefore, bottle-feeding may be the more difficult option.

Often, pediatricians or other providers will recommend to the parents of a tongue-tied baby to simply switch to a bottle to solve the tongue-tie issue nonsurgically. This advice is akin to sweeping the issue under the rug, but sadly, bottle-feeding often does not cure the majority of tongue-tie related issues, except for maternal discomfort. Many of the problems and symptoms are the same as those seen with breastfeeding babies. Visible markers on the lips can include calluses or blisters or even two-tone (outer lip is darker and inner lip is more pale) coloring. These signs come from the baby's need to stabilize and compress the nipple using the lips rather than the tongue, and the constant rubbing/friction creates color changes and calluses or blisters. Often, the upper lip is tucked under while taking a bottle due to the aforementioned reasons or because the lip-tie is so restrictive that the baby physically cannot flange the lip outward to maintain the seal.

> *Bottle-feeding often does not cure the majority of tongue-tie related issues, except for maternal discomfort.*

Babies with poor tongue movement and tongue-tie often exhibit pseudoleukoplakia or "milk tongue," which is the term used when the white of the milk leaves a thick residue on the tongue as the tongue is not able to clear this off of the palate. Often, this can be misdiagnosed as thrush. If the tongue cannot stay cupped on the nipple and is being pulled downward due to restriction, the audible loss of suction is heard in the "clicking" sound associated with ties. This phenomenon can also lead to aerophagia-induced reflux, gassiness, and spitting up frequently, as discussed in previous chapters.

A tongue-tie can also lead to poor lingual grooving and poor overall coordination of the bolus. Poor control and seal can be evidenced by coughing, penetration/aspiration, and liquid leaking out the corners of the mouth (babies may soak through multiple bibs for one feeding). Concerned parents often buy every type of bottle they can find in the hope that one will help their child feed successfully. It is expensive and frustrating for both the parents and the baby!

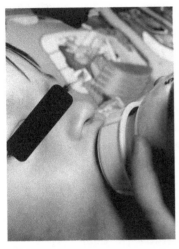
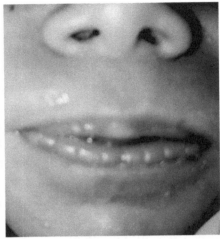

No flange of upper lip   *Lip calluses/compression blisters and two-tone lips*

Without adequate seal and movements, it can take extended amounts of time for a baby to bottle-feed. Parents of babies with ties commonly report during an evaluation that it takes 40 minutes or longer to finish a bottle. While efficient feeding times are dependent on age and the number of ounces consumed, often these babies are burning more calories than they are consuming due to the time and effort exerted to eat. This can lead to poor weight gain or a failure-to-thrive diagnosis. Feeding is literally exhausting for these babies.

This continued negative experience with feeding can impact the baby further in terms of oral aversion and oral developmental experiences. If the baby feels sick or scared (vomiting, coughing, gagging, gas, etc.) every time she eats, she learns that eating is a negative experience and begins to associate oral experiences as such.

It can also directly affect the parents or caregivers of the baby; you can imagine how a mom would feel if she was scared to feed her child due to constant coughing and crying during feedings.

Some tongue-tied babies learn to use their oral structures in an abnormal way to obtain the necessary nutrients they require. These are called compensatory

Feeding is literally exhausting for these babies.

strategies and include using the jaw or cheeks to compress the nipple rather than the tongue-to-palate motion. These patterns are not efficient and often create other maladaptive behaviors, which can lead to poor development of the overall oral-facial complex.[56] There are many techniques that can be used to assist a baby with successful bottle-feeding (tied or not tied), including positioning, changing the type of bottle and/or nipple (shape/flow), pacing, and tactile support. However, in the case of ties, all of these are a band-aid or compensation for being unable to access full oral abilities. When ties are not addressed during this early stage of feeding, future difficulties with eating solids, speech, breathing, and more are often seen.

Cups and Straws

Babies should begin using an open cup between 6 and 9 months of age, depending on development of their oral musculature. Straw drinking is often introduced around 9 months of age, but some babies have demonstrated the ability to master this skill as early as 7 months.[57] Similar to introducing solids, there is a window of time in which a baby may be ready to begin learning this new skill. During this time, developing babies are typically starting to use their tongue, jaw, and lips independently from each other. Whereas a suckle pattern, or front-to-back movement of the tongue, was utilized for bottle and breastfeeding, a true suck pattern begins to emerge around this time and is required for successful cup and straw drinking. This development of the mature swallow pattern starts between 6 and 12 months of age and requires the tip of the tongue to elevate to the alveolar ridge. Cup and straw drinking also require greater activation of the lip muscles. The cup should be stabilized on the lower lip, with the head in a neutral position. If the baby tilts his head back for open cup drinking, he is exposing his airway and risks aspiration or penetration (liquid in the trachea). Similarly, the straw should rest on the center of the lips, and not on the tongue. If the tongue is being used to stabilize the straw or cup, it is a sign that the baby is using the immature suckle pattern to extract the liquid.

Babies with ties sometimes have trouble transitioning to an open or straw cup due to an inability to elevate the tongue tip toward the alveolar ridge and poor use of lip musculature. Additionally, difficulties moving the tongue, jaw, and lips independently of each other inhibit proper function. Often, rather than stabilizing the jaw for cup/straw drinking, the baby will demonstrate an up-and-down jaw motion because the tongue is tethered to the jaw and cannot move by itself.

Often, parents find a cup that "works" for their child, which is usually a spouted sippy cup (different from a straw sippy cup). Spouted sippy cups were designed by an engineer who was tired of his children spilling liquids on the carpet. The cups were not at all designed with oral development in mind, but with fantastic branding and the convenience of a no-spill cup, they quickly became the "go to" after graduating from the bottle. Spouted sippy cups do not encourage the development of the mature swallow pattern, but instead prolong the use of the immature suckle (front to back) pattern. The spout of the sippy cup rests over the anterior portion of the tongue, preventing its elevation to the alveolar ridge, which is why tied babies find these cups to be successful! You could say that spouted sippy cups are another band-aid (and a harmful one at that) for our tied babies. Continued use of these

Continued use of sippy cups can also lead to harmful changes of the orofacial complex, including forward resting tongue posture, open/anterior bite, and mouth breathing.[56]

cups can also lead to harmful changes of the orofacial complex, including forward resting tongue posture, open/anterior bite, and mouth breathing.[56]

Red flags to consider when evaluating this population:
- » Upper lip tucked under during bottle-feeding
- » Clicking sounds during bottle-feeding
- » Extended feeding times (longer than 30 minutes)
- » Falling asleep during bottle-feeds
- » Loss of milk from sides of mouth
- » Pseudoleukoplakia (milk tongue)
- » Lip or compression blisters and/or two-tone lips
- » Excessive jaw excursions and/or cheek dimpling
- » Excessive hiccups, gas or reflux symptoms
- » History of poor breastfeeding skills
- » Inability to hold a pacifier in, or can only take a flat pacifier
- » Collapsing of bottle nipple
- » Coughing with thin liquids from an open or straw cup

Case Study

We recently evaluated a 15-month-old boy who struggled with ear infections, open mouth breathing, excessive drooling, constant congestion, restless sleep, and coughing with thin liquids (water, juice). Mom also reported that he was a poor nurser and was still using a level 1 flow nipple (the slowest flow) for milk in the mornings and night. Mom had attempted a level 2 nipple multiple times throughout infancy, but he coughed with each attempt. He could use a hard spouted sippy cup for thin liquids (spout was long and covered tongue tip), but he coughed with a straw and open cup. After diagnosis of tongue-tie and oral dysfunction due to lingual tethering, he received a lingual frenectomy from a local provider. One week later, he looked like a different child! Congestion had cleared up and mom reported he was sleeping soundly through the night with his mouth closed. He could also now drink from a straw and open cup without coughing. Sippy cups were completely eliminated after the parents learned about their negative consequences. Why could he suddenly use these cups without difficulty? His tongue was able to elevate toward the alveolar ridge to initiate a safe swallow.

One caveat to this success story: This child did not require much follow-up therapy after his procedure, and this is not always the case. Some children need a lot of support following frenectomy to extinguish maladaptive patterns and learn the appropriate ways the tongue and oral structures should function. Some children (often dependent on symptoms and how young they are) bounce back quickly, however, and learn to use their new oral structures almost immediately.

CHAPTER **12**

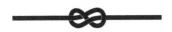

Purees

Megan Musso, MA, CCC-SLP

Introduction to pureed foods generally begins around 6 months of age with signs of readiness. In contrast to breast or bottle-feeding, in which tongue movements are used to extract milk, the lips and jaw are utilized for removing purees from a spoon. This requires more active upper lip movement to meet the spoon and remove the bolus from the spoon, as well as differentiation between jaw, lips, and tongue. A suckle (forward-to-backward) pattern may be used initially with purees, but with time and exposure, a more mature swallow pattern (tongue to alveolar ridge) starts to develop. This pattern begins initially with some elevation of the anterior portion of tongue at about 3 to 4 months, but will not truly mature and reflect an adultlike swallow until the age of 2.

Tied babies often have difficulty with the transition to purees for several reasons. Let's start with the first step in spoon-feeding—removing the food from the spoon. A restrictive labial frenum, or lip-tie, will inhibit the baby from actively using the lip to clear the spoon. In the case of a lip-tie, most of the puree is left on the spoon after a bite. Often, we see parents scrape the puree on baby's upper lip or gum, or "dump" puree into baby's mouth by tipping the spoon upward as they are removing from the mouth. This is a technique that parents used to help baby compensate for the inability to clear the spoon efficiently with active upper-lip movement. It does nothing to help strengthen the labial muscles or encourage them to move independently from the jaw, which we know is critical to future feeding and speech skills as well as development of the orofacial complex.[56,57]

After the puree is transferred to the tied baby's mouth, with or without compensation, the real struggle begins. Often, these babies will use a suckle or tongue thrust pattern (forceful protrusion of the tongue out of the mouth, even though the tongue won't go far because of the tie) to try to swallow the bolus. Can you picture what happens? The bolus immediately spills forward out of baby's mouth as soon as the spoon is removed. Parents often report that they feed the same bite multiple times before the baby actually swallows it. Although this is common when first introducing spoon-feeding as the baby's immature swallow pattern matures into an upward and backward movement, tied babies often do not progress past the suckle pattern. Although some of the bolus may be swallowed with the front-to-back movement of a suckle, most of the bolus will continue to be lost anteriorly.

Another symptom that may present with tied babies is excessive gagging, coughing, and, in extreme cases, choking. When the bolus is placed on the tongue, and the tongue does not elevate to initiate a swallow, gagging occurs. Gagging often results in the forward propulsion of the bolus out of the mouth as well as vomiting. Recurrent negative experiences such as these lead to further oral aversion and panic or frustration for both baby and parents.

"But my baby can take purees from a pouch." I hear this often when taking a case history from parents regarding their child's feeding development. To remove purees from a pouch, what must the child do? Squeeze with his hands and/or suckle. There is no active lip movement involved, and the pouch stays in the mouth during the swallow (much like a bottle). Anterior loss of the bolus would not be seen even if the child is using an

Pouches do not encourage appropriate development of the oral musculature and progression of feeding skills.

120

immature suckle pattern due to the pouch blocking its anterior exit. Pouches are convenient and usually mess-free, which makes them a popular choice for parents on the go; however, these pouches do not encourage appropriate development of the oral musculature and progression of feeding skills. While pouches may be used temporarily for nutritional purposes until oral motor skills are appropriate for spoon feeding, they are not a long-term solution for tolerating purees.

Red flags to consider when evaluating these children:
- » Poor active lip movement to clear spoon (spoon bowl is still full after removal from mouth)
- » Losing food anteriorly during the swallow after multiple exposures
- » Gagging, coughing, or choking
- » Tongue thrust pattern (forceful protrusion of tongue out of the mouth)

CHAPTER 13

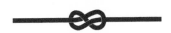

Solids

Megan Musso, MA, CCC-SLP

The transition from purees to solids, meltables, and textured foods is where things really start to get complicated with our tied babies. Up until this point, mom and baby have compensated through various means (great breastfeeding supply, bottle-feeding techniques, scooping/dumping, and using a suckle pattern with purees); however, the art of chewing is a highly complex skill and these techniques are no longer enough.

Soft foods (i.e., those easily chewed or dissolvable) are introduced around 6 to 8 months, along with purees. These foods require baby to use their tongue in new ways, as well as increase independence and coordination of lip, tongue, and jaw movements. Lips and cheeks help stabilize the food, while precise jaw movements are required to bite off a piece of soft food. The transverse tongue reflex causes the tongue to meet the food when placed on the chewing surfaces (gums mostly at this point) for an up-and-down munching pattern. As these foods dissolve quickly in the mouth, a munching pattern is sufficient for chewing. Most often this skill is learned through self-feeding dissolvables such as puffs, Cheerios™, yogurt melts, wafers (which do not necessarily require munching), or easily chewed foods such as pancakes, soft vegetables (sweet potatoes, steamed carrots), and soft cheeses.

There are many ways tied babies are impacted at this stage in development. Most frequently, the major problem is minimal elevation or poor lateral (sideways) movement of the tongue due to a restriction. When a soft-solid, meltable, or anything requiring some type of manipulation (something that cannot be immediately swallowed) is placed on a tied baby's tongue, they will either suck or suckle the food piece until it dissolves, or gag. (Try placing a Cheerio on your tongue and let it sit there for 10 seconds. It doesn't feel good.) Similarly, when placing a meltable laterally in the mouth, the transverse reflex is stimulated; however, tied babies cannot physically move their tongue toward the food to aid in the munching process. If the tongue-tip is anchored down to the floor of the mouth, making it unable to move toward the gums, most children will attempt to reach the food using the sides of their tongue instead.

Melanie Potock, MA, CCC-SLP, an expert in picky eating, describes this inefficiency as moving the tongue like a canoe. "This rocking motion sometimes works," explains Potock, "but is a compensatory method that only helps with very soft, early foods. When the tongue can manipulate just one texture of food, babies learn to stick with that texture, and picky eating is a natural result."[58]

When repeated negative experiences occur with soft solids/meltables, parents begin to avoid giving their children these foods out of fear of coughing, choking, and vomiting. It is also commonly seen at this stage that babies will start to refuse the foods that they are unable to swallow. No self-feeding takes place, as these foods are not tolerated and the jaw musculature does not mature to match the shape and size of foods presented during graded movements. These babies often stay on pureed foods (or graduate from formula to PediaSure®) well into the toddler years before the parents reach out for professional help, at which point there is not only a structural and functional barrier to overcome, but a behavioral one as well. Unfortunately, some of these babies are seen for feeding therapy, but the tongue is not identified as the culprit, and repeated negative experiences with feeding only exacerbate their fear of food.

In summary, here are some red flags to consider when evaluating this population:

> » Gagging, coughing, or choking with textured purees or soft solids after a week of attempts
> » No attempt to self-feed or bring meltables to the mouth
> » Continued use of suckle pattern
> » Tongue thrust or excessive anterior loss of bolus
> » History of poor breastfeeding/bottle-feeding
> » Inability to use a straw or open cup for thin liquids

Case Study

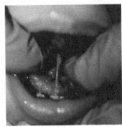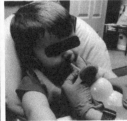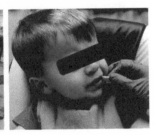

The parents of this 18-month-old boy brought him for an evaluation due to feeding difficulties. He could not tolerate the texture or anything beyond purees and had a very hypersensitive gag reflex. He also suffered from sleep apnea and breathing difficulties. His primary source of nutrition was formula via bottle and some smooth purees. He was unable to use his upper lip to remove puree from the spoon, and a suckle pattern was used to swallow. Textured purees and meltables resulted in vomiting. No attempts to self-feed were noted, and mom reported that he never brought his hands to his mouth during mealtime or play. He was diagnosed with both tongue- and lip-tie after in-depth evaluations of feeding and oral motor skills.

Five days post-frenectomy, mom reported he was sleeping more soundly, but she had not tried textured purees or soft solids. During his first therapy session, a cheese puff was introduced to the lateral gums and his tongue met it at the chew surfaces. A suck/suckle pattern was observed with purees, with huge improvements in active lip movement to clear the spoon. Session 2 resulted in purposeful lateral movement of the tongue with munching on the cheese puff. He also began bringing the puffs to his mouth during this session and was tolerating the small bites he was able to break off with vertical and sometimes diagonal jaw movements. By week 2 of therapy, he was attempting to self-feed smooth purees with a dipping utensil (we use NumNum® pre-spoon GOOtensils™), tolerating purees with texture (homemade guacamole with chunks), biting through cheese puffs with improved jaw movement, and drinking from an open cup and through a straw with some assistance. Removal of the restriction that was inhibiting functional lingual movement allowed this 18-month-old boy to make huge gains in feeding. Although he still has a journey ahead of him to reach age-appropriate skills, he now has access to the structures required to do so.

Table Foods

Between 9 and 12 months of age, the up-and-down munching pattern evolves into a diagonal rotary chew pattern with the addition of purposeful lateral movements of the tongue. This new pattern allows baby to tolerate more adult-like foods, such as casseroles, pastas, soft/chopped meats, vegetables, and fruits. By 1 year of age, a baby should tolerate a safe version of most things on your plate. Soft and squishy foods cut into small pieces that are easy to chew are ideal. They should also be self-feeding some foods at this time, using their tiny fists, fingers or a dipping utensil. These patterns continue to progress over the next year to develop the mature swallow pattern (tongue tip to alveolar ridge for initiation) as well as the rotary (circular) chew pattern, which is required to eat more complex foods, such as meats and raw vegetables.

So what does this mean for tongue-tied babies who are now toddlers? If they experienced any difficulty with breast, bottle-, or spoon-feeding, they will likely have further issues with table foods. On the contrary, some tied toddlers have managed fine up to this point. They compensate for their ties by continuing to use a suck/suckle and munch pattern for soft solids and meltables. Unfortunately, they will continue to use this pattern with complex solids without success.

Let's talk about the first group—our struggling toddlers. These kids will not typically advance to table foods without intervention from a professional. They physically do not have the structures required to manipulate and handle such foods. Until the ties are addressed, these kids will not advance to an age-appropriate diet.

Now let's discuss the group that has compensated well. From the parents' perspective, their child may seem to be functioning adequately— he or she can eat a "variety" of foods; however, when you start asking questions and delving in deeper, the fact that the child is not functioning adequately at all comes to light. When asked which type of foods their child prefers, parents commonly cite what feeding specialist Courtney Gonsoulin, MA, CCC-SLP calls "the white bread diet." These kids like easy-to-chew, quick-to-dissolve foods, such as crackers, soft granola bars, chips, and French fries. They will avoid most meats, although the parents report they eat chicken nuggets. Think about a processed chicken nugget—it requires very little chewing (munching will suffice) and breaks apart in the mouth quite easily. This food is the one type of meat they can handle safely.

These kids have learned to chew their food using the immature munch (up-and-down) pattern. It is not efficient for complex solids; however, if *These kids are slow eaters—it takes a lot more time to munch a food until it is ready to be swallowed when compared with a circular rotary chew.*

you chew up and down long enough, the bolus will eventually be ready to swallow. Clearly, this is an exhausting process. These kids are slow eaters—it takes a lot more time to munch a food until it is ready to be swallowed when compared with a circular rotary chew, which grinds the food quickly. It is commonly reported during evaluation interviews: "My child never finishes his lunch at school," or "He is always the last one at the table."

Let's go back to how exhausting it is to use this munch pattern with complex solids—these kids are often grazers, snacking throughout the day. Why? It is too exhausting for them to eat a complete meal with their immature patterns. Their little bodies can only handle small portions before becoming fatigued and needing a break. These kids are often labeled "picky eaters" because they know which foods are hard for them and avoid them at all costs. The foods they typically avoid include those that scatter in the mouth (breaking into many tiny pieces once bitten into, requiring the tongue to gather from the cheek pockets, etc.), such as corn chips; liquid-solid foods (requiring the child to manage the liquid and skins of solid part simultaneously once bitten into), such as grapes or pineapple; sticky foods (requiring the tongue to remove from the palate, teeth, etc.) such as peanut butter sandwiches; mixed textures (cereal in milk, pasta with sauce); and foods that demand a circular rotary pattern (steak, pizza rolls, firm vegetables, crusty bread).

An efficient chew pattern (circular rotary) requires activation of the cheek muscles with coordinated, rhythmical movements of the jaw. Cheek activation is necessary to keep the food from falling into the sulci (cheek pockets) and remain on the chew surfaces while the tongue works to transfer the food across the midline for symmetrical use of the jaws for chewing. We often see low muscle tone in this population due to inactivity of the cheek musculature secondary to a prolonged munching pattern (picture the adorable 3-year-old who still has "baby cheeks"—watch how he chews). Poor transfer of the bolus across the midline also results in unilateral chew patterns (chewing on one side only), which leads to asymmetrical growth of the jaw musculature.[56] Remember the importance of differentiation of these structures—if a child's tongue is tethered to the floor of her mouth, she physically cannot move it independently of the jaw to use this pattern.

Another observation that is commonly made when evaluating these children is the constant use of water to facilitate a swallow. The tongue is not able to collect the food pieces to bring back to the midline (especially foods that scatter in the mouth) and initiate a mature swallow; therefore, they need water to clear the oral cavity. Some kids even go so far as to "swish and swallow." This should be a red flag to parents and providers. The same lingual movements required to collect and prepare the bolus for swallowing are needed to clean the occlusal surfaces of the teeth. After the swallow, residue (food left behind) is often found in the cheek pockets, on the tongue, and on the occlusal surfaces. These children require multiple swallows per bite of food to clear the oral cavity, which is most certainly exhausting. Water is not the only liquid means to aid swallowing. It is common for kids with ties to drink excessive amounts of milk or juice to fill their bellies and to help wash down any solid foods. When a child drinks milk or juice during meals, he is filling up with liquid and no longer feels hungry. For "picky eaters," this is almost always reported by their parents. Similarly, these kids often drink milk or juice throughout the day, in between meals, and with snacks. Parents struggle with withholding milk because of the additional calories and nutrition it provides; however, when children graze on juice or milk all day, they are typically not ready to eat when meal time comes around.

Tongue-tied children often need liquids to facilitate a swallow.

Pocketing of food in the cheeks or gums is another red flag that a child's oral motor skills are not age-appropriate. While overstuffing the mouth is considered normal until 18 months of age, pocketing is a term used when kids get food trapped in the cheeks or gums. Unfortunately, this is commonly referred to as a behavioral problem, with parents and professionals blaming the child for refusing to swallow his food. In reality, these kids cannot use their tongues to remove the food from the cheek pockets. Remember, cheeks should be active during the chewing process and keep foods from falling into the cheek sulci. Often during a meal, these kids will use their fingers to move food back from the cheek pockets and onto their teeth for chewing or onto their tongue for swallowing. Similarly, food may get trapped in a child's palate (especially if their palate is high); you will see these kids use their fingers to remove the food in order to chew/swallow, which is considered socially inappropriate, but is actually due to poor tongue mobility.

Melanie Potock, MA, CCC-SLP, an expert in picky eating, uses the analogy of a washing machine to describe the forward-backward tongue movement present in this population. "If the child has learned to eat with their lips closed to keep the food in their mouth, the tongue hits the teeth or lips and then rocks back into place to thrust again," explains Potock. "This movement creates a rotation of the food in the mouth, much like a washing machine, making the food go round and round with a tiny bit swallowed as it swishes past the back of the throat. It is an inefficient and exhausting way to eat!"[58]

Red flags to consider when evaluating this population:
- » Limited range of foods; labeled a "picky eater"
- » Limited lingual lateralization to chew surfaces
- » Facilitating swallow with drinking
- » Multiple swallows per bite
- » Problems cleaning teeth surfaces (often history of cavities, dental work)
- » History of poor breastfeeding/bottle-feeding and/or prolonged purees
- » Pocketing of foods
- » Extended feeding times
- » Grazing
- » Unilateral chewing
- » Continued use of suckle or tongue-thrust pattern
- » Poor weight gain

An important note: These symptoms may appear in adults as well. It is not uncommon for an adult who is considering frenectomy due to a reason other than feeding difficulties (i.e., sleep, migraines, speech, breathing, etc.) to exhibit one or more of the above-mentioned symptoms. Often, these patients have compensated using maladaptive patterns and would greatly benefit from oral myofunctional therapy (see Chapter 23) prior to and after frenectomy for optimal results.

Case Study

A 7-year-old boy with a significant history of poor feeding skills, including breastfeeding, bottle-feeding, and transitioning to solids, was evaluated recently at our clinic. His repertoire included foods that were masticated easily (i.e., dissolvables and foods that could be tolerated with a munch pattern). He was referred to our clinic for a functional evaluation after his pediatric dentist identified tongue-tie at a routine checkup. Feeding observation revealed limited-to-no differentiation between jaw, lips, and tongue with a mild tongue thrust swallow pattern. Cues were required to clean oral cavity post-swallow, and he kept his mouth open at rest, with snoring at night. It is worth noting that he had been in speech therapy through the school system for several years due to articulation errors (mainly R production), with minimal progress.

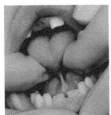 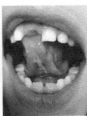 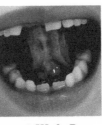 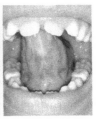

Pre Frenectomy   *1 Week Post*   *2 Weeks Post*   *12 Weeks Post*

When he returned for therapy 7 days post-frenectomy, huge improvements in lingual range of motion were observed; however, these static skills had not carried over into the dynamic movements required for speech and feeding (which is not surprising). Also, as mentioned in previous chapters, there was not only a structural and functional barrier to overcome with feeding, but a behavioral one as well. He had firmly established patterns (the wrong patterns) that had been in use for the past 7 years and had multiple negative experiences when it came to more challenging foods. His treatment plan is lengthy and includes goals as simple as moving the tongue independently from the jaw (something that should have occurred at around 6 to 9 months of age), to establishing a rotary chew pattern, to adding challenging foods (meats, vegetables, etc.) to his preferred food list. He is making huge gains after a few weeks of therapy and has added many new foods to his preferred list, including peanut butter sandwiches and tacos. His jaw movements are more stable and proficient, and his tongue-thrust pattern is almost extinguished; however, he still has a long way to go until he masters age-appropriate and functionally appropriate speech, breathing, and feeding skills.

This child is a great example of how long it takes to extinguish bad habits, eliminate negative associations with foods, and establish new, functional patterns when we wait to treat a tongue-tie. It is hard not to wonder how much of this could have been avoided if he had been released as an infant.

CHAPTER 14

Evaluation, Release, and Aftercare for Children

Richard Baxter, DMD, MS, and Megan Musso, MA, CCC-SLP

To this point, the topics of evaluation, release, and aftercare have focused on infants and babies up to age 1 year. The principles of evaluating, releasing, and healing for a child are similar, but warrant an additional brief chapter for this population and adolescents to adults.

Our clinic (Megan) utilizes The E³ Model, developed by Autumn R. Henning, MS, CCC-SLP, COM for evaluating and treating tethered oral tissues (TOTs).[59] This includes a thorough case history, observations during speech/feeding, formal assessments for speech (articulation, fluency, oral motor), a TOTs-specific evaluation [we use the Hazelbaker Assessment Tool for Lingual Frenulum Function (ATLFF) for infants and the Tongue-Tie Assessment Protocol (TAP) for toddlers to adults], an oral mechanical examination with pictures and descriptors, and a report with discussion of findings as well as recommendations. Conveying findings and recommendations in a parent-friendly way is crucial because often parents and some providers believe that the release alone will fix all of the problems. You should know now that this is not usually the case, and a commitment to therapy following the procedure should be discussed prior to a release. Lastly, the family must select a provider and decide when and how to ensure the best outcome for the patient's release. Why would someone wait to have a release once a tongue- or lip-tie is identified? Most patients require pre-therapy to have the most optimal results regarding a release. Likewise, there are some patients who are too sensitive orally to tolerate the procedure safely. Other reasons may include medical challenges that make the procedure impossible or a parent's inability to commit to aftercare at that time. The decision to move forward with a release once TOTs have been identified should be patient-specific, and the provider must be sensitive to factors that could limit the success for the patient. If you are a provider seeking more information regarding the evaluation and treatment of this population, I highly encourage you to seek out Autumn's course (information can be found in the extra resources chapter at the end of this book).

At our office (Richard), we evaluate children based on a checklist of symptoms and a history taken from the parents. In many cases, the symptoms the child is struggling with are more important than the appearance, which is secondary to the symptoms. With a tether to the tip, there are often significant functional symptoms, but in many cases, less-obvious symptoms may exist as well, such as poor sleep, headaches, neck pain and tension, and increased work during feeding and speaking. It is possible for a child to compensate well with a tongue-tie to the tip, but it is still worth resolving the abnormally tight tissue to see resolution of secondary symptoms. More difficult to diagnose and treat are the posterior tongue-tie varieties.

In our office, we see children for regular dental cleaning visits as well as those referred to us for tongue-tie evaluation. During a routine cleaning, we check the tongue as part of a complete intraoral exam, and often it may appear tighter than normal. However, I would never recommend treatment based on appearance alone. The best option is to ask follow-up questions about feeding, speech, sleep, and nursing issues as a baby. These quick screening questions can lead to a discussion of doing a more thorough examination and history taking (often at a later date so the parent has time to consider whether they are interested based on my recommendation). At this appointment, we evaluate mobility of the tongue and assess for functional deficits using the checklist mentioned above. Many children may appear to have a posterior tongue-tie, but have no symptoms. In these cases, there is nothing to do and no treatment to recommend. If it isn't broke, don't fix it! However, many children do have a posterior tongue-tie and have a lot of symptoms, checking off virtually every box on our diagnostic sheet. Often the tongue appears normal at first glance, so training is key to understanding the multitude of children who could have tongue-tie issues and have flown under the radar up to this point. A child who can still stick out her tongue could still have a posterior tongue-tie and suffer from symptoms with feeding, speech, and sleeping. Thus, protrusion or sticking the tongue out is not a good test to determine the presence of a tongue-tie. Elevation, or lifting the tongue, is the best quick test to screen for tongue-tie. The tongue should elevate freely and be close to or touching the palate when the mouth is maximally opened. Elevation is the key movement for breastfeeding, solid feeding, restful sleep, and speech.

> *Elevation, or lifting the tongue, is the best quick test to screen for tongue-tie.*

Secondary issues that may seem insignificant to some can actually be life-altering, but parents and the child learn to live with extended mealtimes, refusing food, packing food in the cheeks, mumbling, baby talk, slurred speech, and speech delay, and parents may think to themselves, "That's just how kids are sometimes." All the while, there is an underlying issue holding the child back from reaching his full potential, and there is something simple we can do to help him in the development of oral skills and life skills.

The Release

The procedure for releasing a child's tongue is very similar to that of an infant's. We use the same CO_2 laser, similar numbing jelly (although it is stronger and formulated for older children), and often use the same grooved director, if needed. This population now has teeth, so to keep our fingers healthy and intact, a mouth prop, bite block, or "tooth chair" of some kind is needed to stabilize the jaw and allow access to the undersurface of the tongue. We do not routinely—if ever—sedate or put children to sleep for this procedure. That is not typically needed in this population, and using these techniques can save the family from the expense and risk of general anesthesia or sedation.

Using properly prepared assistants, parents (if they wish to participate), and tools, the frenectomy procedure can be performed on anyone—from an uncooperative toddler to a strong, nonverbal, autistic 10-year-old. We position the child in the dental chair, use laser safety glasses, take a before picture with our intraoral camera, and allow the compounded numbing jelly to sit for 5 to 10 minutes. Next, an assistant stabilizes the child's head with the mouth prop in place, and another assistant or a parent holds the child's hands. We begin the 10- to 20-second procedure, vaporizing the tissue of the frenum in a horizontal fashion until we reach the genioglossus muscle and the diamond lays flat without tension. The resulting wound is normally about 1 centimeter wide and only a millimeter or two deep. We then take a postoperative picture and allow the patient to get up out of the chair and have a sugar-free xylitol lollipop if they choose (we are dentists after all!). The procedure is easier and less traumatizing than having a filling done in most cases. The child normally calms down quickly, within a few seconds to a few minutes after the procedure. For more cooperative children, after the jelly numbs the area, we inject a small amount of lidocaine with epinephrine into the frenum to give close to 100% anesthesia of the frenum versus the estimated 90% anesthesia with the topical jelly.

In adolescents and adults, the procedure is the same. Sedation or general anesthesia is not needed for adolescents or adults unless a rare dental phobic patient would benefit from anxiolysis. Nitrous oxide (laughing gas) can be helpful for these cases, or a stronger medicine prescribed by the provider could be used as well. For children through adults, ibuprofen (Motrin® or Advil®) or acetaminophen (Tylenol®) for pain for one to five days is typically sufficient for pain control.

Often parents and patients report results the same day (although some changes take a week or longer). This procedure is not a replacement for speech, feeding, or myofunctional therapy, but should be considered an adjunct to therapy. It is not a magic bullet, but when combined with proper therapy and a team approach, magical things can happen. Better feeding, speech, sleep, and other changes are reported to us at the one-week follow-up. At the one-week follow-up appointment, we often hear that children are speaking new words, speaking more clearly, no longer choking on liquids and foods, eating faster, sleeping less restlessly, waking up more refreshed, and having fewer headaches and less neck pain. And all these changes are stemming from the release of a seemingly insignificant (and sometimes hardly visible) string under the tongue.

Aftercare

Aftercare following frenectomy should be patient-specific. Younger babies might not require much therapy to catch up or learn new skills, while older kids often need more support to help break down bad habits and establish appropriate ones. Treatment plans should be based on the patient's skills and deficits, and there is no "one-size-fits-all" plan. However, one common goal, regardless of the patient's age or symptoms, is to prevent reattachment through the healing phase (3 to 6 weeks, depending on the type of release and child's healing potential). These active wound stretches were discussed in Chapter 8, and I recommend similar stretches for this population as well, although more cooperative children (and older patients) beginning around age 3 can start to do myofunctional exercises.

As previously mentioned, each provider may have a different set of guidelines for helping the wounds heal optimally. Therapy exercises to strengthen the tongue (different from active wound stretching) may include working on lingual range of motion and precision in both static and dynamic movements, specific phonemes or sounds that encourage differentiation or specific movements of the tongue, and exercises to help the jaw, tongue, and lips move independently. Likely, feeding and articulation have been impacted and will also be addressed as appropriate. Again, each patient's therapy plan should be specific to their deficits and skill set. Myofunctional exercises before the procedure and immediately afterward will provide the longest-lasting results. Working with a myofunctional therapist should ideally be a part of every release to retrain the tongue muscles and complex oral patterns to establish normal resting positions and goals of myofunctional therapy. More information about myofunctional therapy can be found in Chapter 23.

CHAPTER 15

———∞———

The Research

Research into the effects of tethered tissues on feeding has not been widely published. It is hard to believe that there is not a single case report in the peer-reviewed literature demonstrating an improvement in solid feeding outcomes after the release of a tongue-tie. It is frustrating for medical and dental professionals who are supposed to base all clinical decisions on "evidence-based" principles, because the literature is lacking in this area. Almost every day, providers who release tongue-ties see improvements in children's feeding, and occupational therapists and speech therapists report the same thing.

When a release is performed on an appropriately selected patient using the "best practices" put forth in this book, there is a very good chance that the patient will see improvement. The only questions that remain are how much improvement will occur, and how quickly the improvement will be evident. It is important for parents and providers not to miss opportunities for establishing normal feeding and speech in children who are facing challenges. The best care results when a team-based approach is used to address each child's needs.

There is a growing body of collective knowledge of many practitioners as to what works, which is summarized here. It is our hope that in the near future, larger series of cases and short-term randomized controlled trials will help to answer any questions that remain about the science supporting these methods.

In this new millennium, the use of conferences, social media, and other forms of communication between clinicians facilitates the spread of knowledge in new ways. Today's parents of young infants are accustomed to accessing the most up-to-date information available, right along with their providers. There are varying lengths and types of aftercare stretches and exercises, and there are different therapies available for parents to utilize before and after the release. How practitioners and parents piece together an individual child's unique care is the artistic side of diagnosis and treatment. Medicine, dentistry, and allied health professions all marry art and science to varying degrees. Effective approaches to any clinical problem use the science to achieve a foundation on which to build a work of art to help a particular child and family.

Silva et al. (2009)

A study by Brazilian researchers Silva et al. looked at chewing patterns in patients with altered lingual frena.[60] They noticed some differences in chewing in a cross-section of 10 patients with normal lingual frena and 10 patients with altered lingual frena. The patients ranged in age from 12 to 25 years old. They noted that patients with altered frena were 5.4 times more likely to have altered tongue mobility than those with normal frena. When they observed the chewing patterns of the patients, 100% of the normal frena patients chewed with their posterior teeth, whereas only 47% of the patients with altered lingual frena chewed with their posterior teeth. The other 53% used their tongue to knead the food or used their anterior teeth to chew. Finally, they noted that when people with altered lingual frena chewed, they were 5.7 times more likely to use atypical muscle patterns than those with normal lingual frena. This article does not delve into feeding of children specifically, although it is helpful to have it documented (even with a small sample size) that chewing is impacted negatively by a tongue-tie.

Baxter and Hughes (2018)

When the first paragraph of this chapter was composed, there were no published case reports describing solid feeding improvements after tongue-tie releases in children. Therefore, two of the authors (Baxter and Hughes) working on this project, who see results daily, decided to submit a series of five cases to the *International Journal of Clinical Pediatrics*. Now, several months later, the article, "Speech and Feeding Improvements in Children after Posterior Tongue-Tie Release: A Case Series," has been published.[61] This article is open access, meaning we paid to allow anyone to access the full text and PDF of the article to share with others free of charge. In this article, five cases that show dramatic improvements in speech, feeding and sleep are presented. All were released with the CO_2 laser and patients performed stretches for 3 weeks afterward. The cases are summarized below.

Case 1

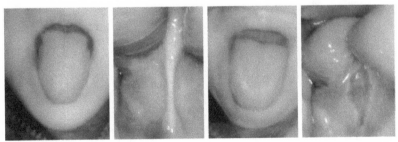

Before Protrusion   Before Elevation   After Protrusion   After Elevation

A 5-year-old boy was referred for trouble with speech and feeding. He struggled with L, TH, S, R, and M sounds, which worsened as he talked faster. He spoke softly and mumbled often, and was shy and not confident in communicating with others. He was a picky eater and gagged on foods of various textures, especially on mashed potatoes. He had trouble with purees as a baby, and slept restlessly. When examined, he could stick his tongue out to about a third of the way down his chin, but he was unable to elevate his tongue to get close to his palate. He had a posterior Kotlow Class II tongue-tie presenting as a thick band of tissue holding his tongue down, but it was hidden from view.

He received laughing gas (nitrous oxide), a small amount of lidocaine was injected into the frenum, and all of the restricting fibers were released using a CO_2 laser. No sutures were used, and no bleeding occurred, and immediate gains in tongue elevation and protrusion were visible. Immediately after the procedure, his mother noticed clearer speech, and he was able to say S and M sounds better. He also gagged less and tried foods he had refused before, including pork and quiche.

Case 2

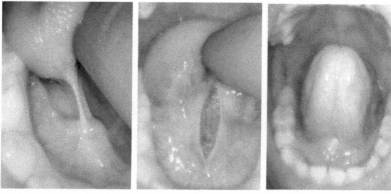

Before Elevation   *After Elevation*   *Healing at 1 Week*

This 5-year-old boy had trouble with S, R, and CH sounds. He gagged and vomited when eating certain textures, and he avoided new foods. He also complained frequently of neck pain. This child also had a difficult-to-observe and diagnose Kotlow Class II posterior tongue-tie.

He was given nitrous oxide and a small amount of lidocaine into the frenum, and 10 seconds later the restricted fibers were vaporized with no bleeding or sutures, leaving a diamond-shaped wound. At one week, he had no pain, he showed increased elevation, and his mother, a physical therapist, reported that he enjoyed an increased range of motion in his neck, which allowed him to sleep more comfortably. He was easier to understand and could now say S, R, and CH much more clearly. He took larger bites of food and now could eat yogurt, potatoes, pudding, and cake without gagging or spitting up. Previously, his mother said, he would not have tolerated these foods.

Case 3

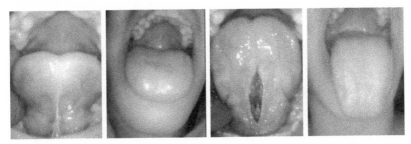

Before Elevation   Before Protrusion   After Elevation   After Protrusion

This 11-year-old girl used baby talk, stuttered, mumbled, and had trouble with TH and L sounds. As a baby, she had difficulty nursing, a poor latch, colic, and trouble gaining weight. When she began eating solids, she was very picky and ate slowly. She complained of neck pain daily and nighttime teeth grinding (bruxism). She was also a habitual mouth breather, and had chronic sinus infections. Her palate was narrow with a high arch. She had a Kotlow Class II posterior tongue-tie and could stick her tongue out to just past her lips, but not much farther.

After a 20-second procedure that she tolerated well with no reported pain, she had significantly improved elevation and protrusion of her tongue. After the procedure, her mother reported she was easier to understand and could make speech sounds she previously could not make. Remarkably, she had immediate relief from neck tension and pain. During a phone call 3 weeks after the procedure, the mother reported that her daughter had significantly better speech and more appropriate food intake. She was eating full meals consistently, and had improved quality of sleep.

Case 4

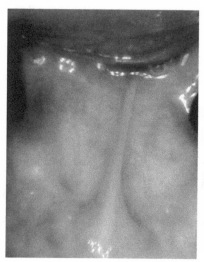 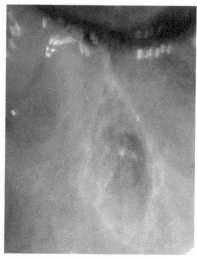

Before Elevation   *After Elevation*

A 2-year, 10-month-old boy was referred because he was making minimal progress in speech therapy. He did not begin babbling until 2 years of age and currently had around 30 words, indicating a speech delay. His speech was difficult for his parents and outsiders to understand. He packed food in his cheeks like a chipmunk and had a history of recurrent ear infections. His posterior Kotlow Class I tongue-tie was barely visible, and looked like a thin string (see picture) that seemed inconsequential.

With only some lidocaine/prilocaine jelly used for anesthesia, he had some discomfort during the procedure, but calmed down immediately afterward. His tongue elevation improved immediately, and the area now felt soft and spongy with normal elasticity. He also performed exercises and stretches for 3 weeks. At the 1-week follow-up appointment, his mother reported he now was babbling most of the day, was saying new words, and even combining words into short phrases, such as "Up me," which he had never previously done. He also began making animal sounds. He seemed less frustrated overall and was a happier child. Although his feeding wasn't mentioned as a concern before the correction, he was now eating a lot more and eating his food much faster than previously, and he also stopped packing food in his cheeks.

Case 5

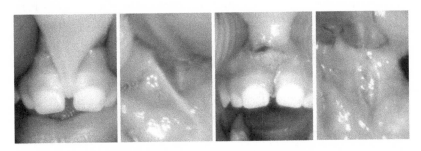

A 17-month-old girl had speech and language delays. She began babbling at 15 months old and only had a few words, such as "mama" and "dada." Her pediatrician and GI specialist recommended an upper GI scope and modified barium swallow due to a history of digestive and swallowing issues, including frequent choking on liquids. As a baby, she suffered from a poor latch on bottle and breast, poor weight gain, reflux, and colic. Nursing was very painful for her mother. Mom also reported that it was difficult to brush her upper teeth, and she slept restlessly, awakening frequently during the night. She was examined and diagnosed with a significant Kotlow Class IV lip-tie and posterior Kotlow Class II tongue-tie. Numbing jelly and a few drops of lidocaine were injected into the lip- and tongue-ties.

The lip-tie was lasered for around 15 seconds at 1.45 avg W with the CO_2 laser, and the tongue-tie was lasered for only 5 seconds. No sedation of any kind was used. Immediate gains in mobility and elevation were noted. Her mother stated that immediately after the procedure, her daughter said four new words: "bubba," "pawpaw," "juice," and "hot." The same day of the procedure, she also stopped choking on liquids and spitting up, with no further choking or vomiting episodes. Her mother also reported that the quality of her voice improved and was "louder, clearer, and not as raspy."

These stories are a testament to the functional issues caused by the anatomical restrictions of tongue-ties in older babies, toddlers, and children. Most children see improvement after the releases, but sometimes it takes several days to weeks and the help of intensive therapy to overcome compensations. Other times it is immediate and the children instinctively know what they need to do, and their reflexes are totally intact; after the release they quickly achieve normal function. It is our hope that these 5 recently reported cases will inspire future research by additional clinicians. Children with posterior tongue-ties can go years before the restriction is identified. However, the pieces of the puzzle are becoming easier to see, and there is hope that increasing numbers of children with similar presentations will be identified, examined, and receive proper treatment to help them resolve these life-altering deficits, not only in feeding and speech, but, as we'll explore later, other related challenges.

Section 3: Speech

Many of the same structures are used for both speech and feeding, so it is no surprise that many children who have issues with feeding may also exhibit speech errors. Coordination of a variety of oral structures along with adequate air flow is required for speech sound production. The tongue is the most versatile and commonly used articulator. The tongue has a limited range of motion when a tongue-tie is present, which can affect its ability to reach various placement points in the mouth to produce different speech sounds. Limited range of motion can also affect oral resonance, which is a vital part of speech production. In this section, we explore how oral structures interact with each other to produce speech, and how a tongue-tie can affect the relationship between these structures.

CHAPTER 16

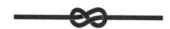

How Do We Produce Speech?

Lauren Hughes, MS, CCC-SLP

The production of speech sounds is complicated work. Structures in the mouth, called articulators, are used to direct airflow and create resonance. There are 44 speech sounds (i.e., phonemes) in the English language. All 44 sounds are produced using varying combinations of these articulators. For example, D and G sounds are both produced by pressing the tongue against the palate, but different parts of the tongue and palate are used for each sound. The placement of these articulators allows air flow and resonance to be altered so different sounds can be produced. Speech is one of the most sophisticated fine-motor functions in the body. In this chapter, we'll examine speech sound production in greater detail and identify the structures required to produce speech sounds. In the next chapter, we'll talk more in depth about how the presence of a tongue-tie can affect the production of speech sounds.

As one of the most sophisticated fine-motor functions in the body, speech production requires several systems to work together. These systems include articulation (placement of articulators), oral resonance (the manipulation of airflow), voicing (use of the vocal cords), and fluency (the rate and smoothness of speech). Let's break down each of these systems and discuss them in more detail.

Components of Speech Production

Articulation

According to the *Oxford Living Dictionary*,[62] articulation is defined as, "The formation of a speech sound by constriction of the air flow in the vocal organs at a particular place and in a particular way." Merriam-Webster[63] defines articulation as "the action or manner in which the parts come together at a joint."

The word *articulation* is used in the medical field to describe how two bones come together to form a joint (e.g., knee, shoulder, elbow). It is also used in construction to describe various materials (e.g., brick, concrete) that come together in a certain way. For our purposes, and likely the most common use of "articulation," we cover how oral structures come together to create speech sounds. Now that we know "articulation" means "two parts coming together," we need to know what those "parts" are when talking about speech production. Some oral structures are static, whereas others are dynamic (in motion). The primary oral structures used for articulation include:

» Alveolar ridge (static)
» Lips (dynamic)
» Tongue (dynamic)
» Hard palate (static)
» Soft palate (dynamic)
» Teeth (static)
» Jaw (dynamic)

Each structure has a role in the production of speech. Let's take a closer look at these oral structures to see how each functions.

Alveolar Ridge: The alveolar ridge is the raised area you feel behind your top front teeth. While the alveolar ridge is static and does not move, it is an important placement point for the tongue to create a variety of sounds, including D, T, N, and L. Say the sounds mentioned previously and notice how your tongue "taps" or rests against the alveolar ridge.

Lips: The lips are used together and separately to create different speech sounds. For example, the F sound is made by placing the upper teeth against the bottom lip, whereas B is made by pressing both lips together. Say the word "boom." Notice how your lips press together and round while you say the word.

Tongue: The tongue is the most versatile and most commonly used articulator. It is used in every speech sound in some way. For sounds like B or M, it rests at the bottom of the mouth to create a larger oral resonance chamber. The tongue raises and lowers to create different vowel sounds. Different parts of the tongue touch the teeth, alveolar ridge, hard palate, and soft palate to create different consonant sounds. Say the sounds G (like "guitar"), S, and CH (like "chew"). Notice how different parts of your tongue interact with different areas of your mouth.

Hard Palate: The hard palate is what we call the "roof of the mouth." This is the flat, bony structure that fills most of the area between your upper teeth. It also forms the floor of the nose. The hard palate is static and doesn't move, but plays an important role in creating oral resonance for the production of different sounds. Depending on the structure of the hard palate, some speech sounds can be difficult to produce or sound distorted. The hard palate is often high and narrow in children and adults who have a tongue-tie due to a low resting tongue posture while swallowing.[64] Tongue-tied babies are born with a high palate from low posture during swallowing in utero as well. Breastfeeding, tongue-tie release, myofunctional exercises, palatal expanders, and functional orthodontic appliances all help to broaden the palate.

Soft Palate: This is the soft area behind the hard palate that also allows air to pass from the nose into the throat and to the airway.

The back of the tongue meets the soft palate and hard palate to create sounds such as K and G. The soft palate is also important in creating sounds such as M and N, which are produced by directing air through the nose. Say the sounds K (like "kick") and M. You should feel the back of your tongue raise to say "kick," and you may feel your soft palate elevate to say M.

Teeth: Our teeth are static and therefore don't move during speech production, but they play a role in oral resonance. You may have noticed this when a child loses a front tooth and tries to say the S sound or when a person removes his or her dentures. Their speech sounds different than when all their teeth are in the appropriate place. The teeth also play a role in sounds such as TH (like "this" or "tooth"). When you make this sound, notice how your tongue slides between your teeth.

Jaw: The jaw is used for all speech sounds in some way. Most often, it moves up and down to create a wide or narrow oral cavity to change oral resonance, and provides support when moving the tongue. It also provides stability for the oral cavity as a person combines speech sounds to make phrases and sentences. Say the words "ouch," "meet," and "cake." Notice how your jaw moves as you produce the different sounds in each word.

Oral Resonance

Oral resonance was mentioned several times already, but let's talk about it in more depth. Think about a sailboat. If the sail is moved just slightly one way or another, the boat will move in a different direction. Articulators can be viewed in a similar way. The smallest movement of an articulator can result in the production of a different sound. Another way to think about it is how the air goes around a car as it moves. The car "displaces" the air and makes it behave differently than the way it would behave if the car was not there.

Oral resonance is a combination of air being exhaled and articulators manipulating that air to make different sounds. The production of each speech sound varies based on the amount of interference created by the tongue, lips, and teeth. It is further affected by how open the mouth is (jaw) and the shape/structure of the hard and soft palates. If the hard palate has a high arch or the soft palate doesn't elevate at the right time, a speech sound may come out distorted or sound more like a different speech sound.

Voicing and Air Supply

Another level of complexity is whether a speech sound is voiced or voiceless. A voiced sound occurs when the vocal cords are pressed together as air is moved past, whereas the vocal cords remain still and open when a voiceless sound is produced. For example, the sounds T and D are made in the same way, by tapping the tongue against the alveolar ridge (the raised section of the hard palate directly behind the top teeth). The only difference in the production of these two sounds is whether or not the vocal cords are used. Let's do a hands-on activity to better understand this concept. Place your hand on your throat and say the words "toe" and "doe." You should feel a vibration in your throat when you say "doe" because the vocal cords are used to produce the D sound. You can repeat this exercise with words like "bye" and "pie" or "cake" and "gate." You should feel a vibration in your throat with "bye" and "gate," since the vocal cords are used for B and G.

Fluency

Fluency is the smoothness or "prosody" of speech. For the purposes of this book, let's talk about a person's ability to talk at a fast or slow rate while maintaining smooth speech. We've seen that the production of even one speech sound involves several different actions and structures. Combining sounds into words and sentences requires a certain level of coordination. It is difficult to maintain the necessary coordination when oral structures are not working properly. Articulators must be able to move freely or be formed correctly to allow for proper coordination. If the tongue, for example, is not able to move freely to different areas of the mouth, coordination is limited and could result in variations in speech, including sound or word repetitions and a slow rate of speech.

Common Articulation Errors

In the next chapter, we'll address speech sound disorders that are related to tongue-ties. What follows is a brief description of the types of speech sound errors so we can discuss further in the next chapter:

> *Substitutions:* when a speech sound is replaced by another speech sound. Common substitutions include T for K, D for G, W for R, and Y for L. For example, the word "cat" becomes "tat" or "yellow" becomes "yeyow."

> *Distortions:* a speech sound is replaced by something other than one of the 44 English phonemes. Some examples include the S sounding "slushy" or the presence of a lisp.

> *Omissions:* when a speech sound is missing from a word. A child may say "bi" for "big" or "pen" for "open."

> *Additions:* speech sounds are added to words when they shouldn't be. Examples include "buhlack" instead of "black" or "catuh" instead of "cat."

Conclusion

The purpose of this chapter was to illustrate the complexity of speech production and the system of structures that work together to produce even a single word. When an oral structure does not function in an adequate manner, the production of speech becomes difficult. In the next chapter, we will discuss how the structural abnormality of a tongue-tie can affect speech production.

CHAPTER 17

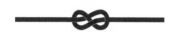

Tongue-Ties and Speech

Lauren Hughes, MS, CCC-SLP

Think about a child who has lost a front tooth. Some speech sounds are going to sound different until the adult tooth comes in. This is a minor and temporary structural change that alters the way speech sounds. What happened the last time you had a cold? Your voice probably sounded different because the airflow between the throat and the nose was blocked due to mucus or swelling. For those few days you were sick, the soft palate and airway were not functioning properly, so your voice continued to sound strange until the mucus and swelling returned to normal.

These are examples of temporary structural issues that affect speech quality. Tongue-ties are permanent structural issues that may affect speech quality. There is no evidence that a tie can be stretched or altered using exercises or therapy alone, so surgical revision is the only known treatment for a restricted frenum. Speech therapy is often required before and/or after the release to modify oral motor behaviors and teach the child how to correctly produce speech sounds. While speech therapy is a vital part of the process, it can't make a tongue-tie disappear. Therefore, it is important that a speech-language pathologist and the release provider work closely to provide the best care for the patient.

When my brother and I were little, we would tie our dad's shoelaces together when he was taking a nap. Usually he would notice before standing up, but once or twice we were tricky enough to make him trip or stumble when he stood up. (Kids can be mean, right?) A tongue-tie is a lot like having your shoelaces tied together.[59] With a tie, the tongue has trouble moving separately from other oral structures, such as the jaw, or reaching placement for speech sounds (i.e., alveolar ridge, soft palate). With the information learned in the previous chapter in mind, let's explore how a tongue-tie affects speech production and why the release of the tether can improve the quality of speech.

Speech Production Components

Articulation

As discussed in the previous chapter, articulation requires several oral structures to work together. The tongue is arguably the most important structure in the articulation system. If movement of the tongue is restricted, it has difficulty in reaching the placements required for producing sounds. Depending on the severity and location of the restriction, a person may not be able to raise the back of their tongue to create the K and G sounds, or have difficulty coordinating their tongue muscles to make L and R.

Oral Resonance

Oral resonance requires that the oral cavity be a certain size and shape according to which sound is being produced. The presence of a tongue-tie can cause speech sounds to be distorted (see previous chapter for a definition of distortion). These errors often follow a pattern. For example, it is common for children to replace K and G with T and D. Distortions can be caused by imprecise placement of articulators or by altered oral resonance. Have you ever seen children sit in front of a fan and make sounds or say words? They love it because it sounds silly and different than their "normal" voice. Altered oral resonance is similar. When the airflow coming from the lungs is directed or restricted in a different way, the sounds a person produces will also sound different. A tongue-tie may restrict the tongue from moving in a way to direct airflow properly.

Voicing and Air Supply

While a tie does not directly affect voicing or air supply, it stands to reason that it adds stress to the load of speech production. If you're like me, taking groceries into the house in one trip is a goal to be accomplished. On the days I spend way too much money at the store, I just can't manage those last few bags or that big bag of dog food. I know that one more item added to the load would mean dropping the jar of salsa and having to clean it up. Having a tongue-tie or other oral motor disorder can cause a similar "overloading." When a person has to concentrate on coordinating his or her tongue rather than it being an automatic movement, it may impact the ability to focus on voicing or use all of the airflow efficiently. This is an uncommon but possible symptom of a tie.

Fluency

Fluent speech requires the tongue to move efficiently and smoothly. When the tongue is restricted by a tongue-tie, it can feel as if the tongue is weighed down. Think about a time that you lifted weights. If you used weights that were a little too heavy, your arms moved slower and may have started to shake. If you had weights strapped around your wrists, it would be harder to do fine motor tasks such as tying your shoes or writing. The weights would restrict your movements and decrease coordination. A tie can cause the same type of incoordination and inefficiency, which could cause stuttering. When a person with a tongue tie talks fast or for extended periods of time, fluent speech can be even more difficult to maintain.

Is a Tongue-Tie Affecting My Child's Speech?

Now that we've talked about how a tongue-tie can affect speech, let's look at some speech-related symptoms that can be caused by a tie. This list is by no means exhaustive, and your child doesn't need to have all the symptoms for a tongue-tie to be affecting his or her speech.[59]

» Frustration with communication
» Poor speech intelligibility in connected speech (e.g., phrases, sentences, conversation)
» Strange errors (e.g., frequent distortions or errors that are uncommon)
» Stuttering
» Slow and/or slurred speech
» Apraxic-like speech:
  • Inconsistent speech sound errors (e.g., may say "fen" for pen, then say "ben" for pen on the next repetition)
  • Voicing errors (e.g., "down" for "town" or "ped" for "bed")
  • Placing stress on syllables incorrectly ("BUH-nan-uh" instead of "buh-NAN-uh")
» Errors with vowel sounds
» Avoids certain words or speaking situations
» Speech delays or disorders, particularly errors with the following speech sounds:
  • K, G, and NG (e.g., si**ng**)
  • SH, CH, DGE (e.g., **edge**), Y (i.e., **y**es)
  • TH (e.g., too**th** or **th**ose)
  • T, D, N, L, R, S, Z

Although it is likely that your child has a tongue-tie if several of these symptoms are present (especially with a history of nursing issues as a baby, or if you also see feeding and/or sleep problems), remember that there could be many potential causes for these errors. It is important to have your child evaluated by a speech-language pathologist (SLP) who has experience with tongue-ties, oral motor disorders, and speech sound disorders. The SLP can determine the cause(s) of speech errors and make sure all areas of concern are addressed as needed.

A word of caution about the potential results of a tongue-tie release procedure: Parents and their children typically notice some improvement in speech, feeding, or sleep post-procedure. However, some families observe minimal-to-no changes in these behaviors after a tongue-tie has been released. Limited results can be expected when a release is incomplete and restricted tissue is still present. Parents and medical professionals alike should also acknowledge the possibility of other causes that are contributing to the continued presence of symptoms. Consider the following scenario:

Brittany is a picky eater, and others have a hard time understanding her speech. Her diet is limited to foods such as pizza, French fries, yogurt, and chicken nuggets. She is very reluctant to try new foods and often has a strong emotional reaction when prompted to try something new. When her parents listen to her speech closely, they noticed she is unable to say sounds such as T, D, K, G, SH, and S. They take her to an SLP for an evaluation, who notices the presence of a tongue-tie. The SLP refers Brittany to a pediatric dentist who agrees with the diagnosis and performs the release procedure. At her one-month follow-up with the dentist, Brittany's speech is a little clearer, but no changes are noted in her eating habits. When they next see the SLP, she performs another oral motor exam and asks Brittany's parents more questions about the speech and feeding symptoms. Parents report that mornings are often a fight in their home because getting dressed is such an ordeal. Brittany needs her socks to be positioned just so, and any tags must be removed from clothes before she will wear them. The SLP determines that Brittany has a sensory processing disorder that causes her to reject certain food textures. She also notices that Brittany developed a few "bad habits" over the years to compensate for limited tongue movement. The SLP recommends treatment for a feeding and oral motor disorder, as well as occupational therapy to address other sensory needs.

While Brittany did have a tongue-tie that needed to be released, she and her family did not see immediate results due to the presence of other contributing factors. Continued intervention by the SLP and other medical professionals helped this family find answers to help Brittany develop appropriate feeding and speech skills. This scenario lays the foundation for what we will discuss for the remainder of this chapter, which includes the role of speech therapy in the tongue-tie release process, and the presence of compensatory strategies and contributing factors.

Speech Therapy: Before and After

Speech therapy before and after a release procedure is important for several reasons. Therapy before the procedure can help prepare the child and family for the procedure and aftercare activities. Parents and children have a chance to practice any prescribed stretches, exercises, or activities so they are comfortable with the process before a wound is present in the mouth. Reattachment of the restriction is common in children who do not participate in aftercare as prescribed, so pre-therapy can decrease instances of reattachment.

A speech-language pathologist should be following your child and can make recommendations for appropriate treatment after the procedure. Children with mild speech sound disorders may only require a few therapy sessions to correct speech errors. However, the presence of restricted lingual frenulum can create other problems that need to be addressed through speech therapy. These children often present with oral motor or feeding disorders in addition to speech sound errors. By releasing the tongue tie, oral motor and speech disorders can be more easily corrected through speech therapy. It's important to remember that releasing the tongue tie will not magically cure a child's symptoms, but it can be an important step along the journey to better speech.

Conclusion

The presence of a restricted frenum under the tongue can contribute to speech delays and disorders. Depending on when the tongue-tie is discovered and treated, children will have varying degrees of speech symptoms. Some children may have little-to-no symptoms related to speech production, but they may compensate for the restriction by producing sounds in ineffective ways. These compensations and structural changes caused by a tie, such as a high or narrow palate, poor tongue resting posture, and others, can cause issues down the road, such as neck and back tension, temporomandibular joint (TMJ) disorders, and frequent sinus infections. Just because a child doesn't have speech or feeding symptoms doesn't mean the tongue-tie shouldn't be released. Parents should work closely with their potential release provider, SLP, and other team members to make the best decision for their child. Whether or not improvements are observed post-procedure, remember that other factors could be contributing to continued speech or feeding symptoms. Consultation with an SLP and other relevant team members can help ensure all areas of need are addressed through speech therapy or other needed services.

CHAPTER 18

The Research

When it comes to tongue-tie research, it seems that the babies receive all the attention. Certainly, nursing is critical and tongue-tie release can impact nursing in significant ways, but when babies grow up with uncorrected restricted tongues, a whole host of other issues can arise. We need research to guide our clinical decisions for these older children. There is a dearth of research relating to feeding and tongue-ties, but thankfully there are a few peer-reviewed articles relating to speech and tongue-ties.

Messner and Lalakea (2002)

Messner and Lalakea performed a prospective study of 30 children with tongue-tie (from ages 1 to 12 years) to identify any differences noted after their releases.[65] This study included speech evaluations, but they weren't standardized. The children were told to perform tongue exercises for one month after the procedure. It should be noted that 26 of the 30 children in this study were treated under general anesthesia, and there were no surgical complications in any of the children. The study included a subset of 21 patients, who underwent a formal speech evaluation before the procedure. Of those, 15 patients (71%) were found by the speech-language pathologists (SLPs) to have articulation errors caused by the decreased mobility of the tongue. A smaller subset of 15 children was evaluated before and after the procedure by their SLPs (12 different diagnosticians), and of these 15 children, 11 had abnormal articulation before the procedure. Nine of these 11 patients improved after the procedure—an 82% success rate. In the other two patients, tongue mobility improved, but articulation was still a struggle. However, 1 of the 2 patients was very young and hard to evaluate. The parents also noted a difference in speech (p < 0.01), and they were very happy with the tongue-tie release procedure overall. The authors make several points in the article that are worth sharing:

> » Tongue protrusion is not the best criterion to use when predicting whether or not a child needs tongue-tie release.
> » The inter-incisal distance (elevation of the tongue with the mouth open) is a better test of tongue restriction than tongue protrusion.
> » Significant gains in mobility and articulation can be found after a tongue-tie release, which is a minor procedure with very few risks.
> » Speech sounds that are affected are T, D, Z, S, TH, N, and L.
> » It is difficult to know which children with tongue-ties will develop speech issues.

These findings and recommendations should be heeded and implemented in clinical practice. When people say that tongue-ties do not affect speech, what they should really say is that tongue-ties don't always affect speech articulation. We have seen patients with tongue-ties to the tips of their tongues who have perfect articulation. However, they still struggle with speaking rapidly and loudly, or get tired when speaking, because they must exert tremendous effort to

Significant gains in mobility and articulation can be found after a tongue-tie release, which is a minor procedure with very few risks.[65]

speak. Having a tongue-tie is like trying to walk with a rubber band around one's legs. It can be done, but it takes much more effort.

Some children have what appear to be tongue-ties, but no issues with speech at all. So in this case, if inquiries about secondary speech, feeding, and sleep issues are made, and there are still no concerns, then there is nothing to be done. As we've said all along, "If it ain't broke, don't fix it!" But for children with speech issues, especially those involving the known tongue-tie sounds and for children with histories of nursing and feeding issues, tongue-ties should be at the TOP of the list of the differential diagnoses. A sneaky posterior or submucosal tongue-tie is likely to blame. This article mentioned that the authors planned to have a control group, but all of the parents strongly preferred for their children to have the procedures and not wait until later. One possibly faulty conclusion that is mentioned in this article regards speech delay. The article states that tongue-ties do not cause speech delay; however, the study was not designed to address speech delay, so this statement is not evidence-based. In children with speech delays and tongue-ties— often posterior—we have noticed that once the ties are released, many patients begin babbling and talking more, either the same day or within a few days! There are no publications supporting this observation, but common sense suggests that children who have difficulty producing sounds are likely to be discouraged from using language.

Ito et al. (2015)

This article by Ito et al. (2015) is from a Japanese group of researchers and describes 5 children ages 3 to 8 years who were given an articulation test of 50 pictures in Japanese and were graded by a speech therapist.[66] The results before and after were compared at 1 month, 3 months, and 1 to 2 years. They noticed that the children used substitutions (saying another sound for the correct sound), omissions (leaving out a sound within a word), and distortions (lisping, muffling, etc.) when speaking. The children were treated under general anesthesia in 4 cases and 1 case was clipped in the clinic. Most of the problems were with the sounds S, T, D, and R. Four patients collectively utilized 19 substitutions before the procedure, which decreased to 10 by 1 month after the procedure, 7 at 3 to 4 months afterward, and only 1 substitution in 1 patient by 1 to 2 years after the procedure. Five omissions before the procedure decreased to 3 at 1 month, 2 at 3 to 4 months, and 1 in only 1 patient at 1 to 2 years after the procedure. These are highly significant findings. Thirteen distortions were observed in 5 patients before the procedure, and that decreased to 8 at 3 to 4 months, but increased to 1 at 1 to 2 years afterward. One patient out of the 5 accounted for the entire increase in distortion at the 1 follow-up. All of the other patients (80%) decreased their observed distortions. This study used a standardized articulation test that was able to distinguish between the child's speech before and after the procedure, and they noted that substitutions and omissions improved relatively early after the procedure. They reasoned that distortions, which are more minor than substitutions and omissions, take longer to improve, but this finding was based on 1 patient's distortion becoming worse. It seems that the release is, in fact, helpful and does improve speech, but just as all children are different, the amount it will help each child is different as well.

Walls et al. (2014)

This study surveyed hospital records of 3-year-old children to discern whether the children who had tongue-ties at birth and had them clipped via frenotomy had better speech than those who never had them corrected.[67] This study was attempting to answer the question: "Does clipping a baby's tongue-tie set them up for better speech in the future?" Seventy-one children who had a frenotomy or clip done in the hospital shortly after birth comprised the surgical intervention group. This group was compared with a group of 15 children who had a tongue-tie but no frenotomy, and a third control group of 18 who never had a tongue-tie. The results of this study showed that the children who had their tongue-tie clipped at birth had better speech outcomes 3 years later than the group of children who did not have their tongue-tie clipped. The children who had it clipped had the same speech outcomes as the children who had never had a tongue-tie. In addition, the children in the group that did not have their tongue-ties released had more difficulty cleaning their teeth with their tongues, licking the outsides of their lips, and eating ice cream.

Dollberg et al. (2011)

This study attempted to answer the same question as the previous study by comparing children who had tongue-ties treated during early infancy (8 children), to children with untreated tongue-ties (7 children), and a control group with no tongue-tie history (8 children).[68] They discovered that the children who were treated for tongue-ties with a frenotomy or clip as infants made fewer speech errors than children who did not have their tongue-ties clipped. However, the group of children who were clipped still had more errors than the group of children who had no tongue-ties at all. The children with tongue-ties had more trouble moving their tongues than the control group or the group that were clipped as infants. Why did the children who had their tongue-ties clipped continue to exhibit speech errors? The authors hypothesize that the depth of the frenotomy or "clip" may have been inadequate in these children, and, as a result, the children still had residual restriction of tongue movement interfering with their speech. It is likely that variability in the techniques used to relieve the restricted tissues may have confounded the data set in this study. It is not uncommon for babies and older children with previous clips to continue to have issues because they were not released deeply enough. When this occurs, a second procedure is usually necessary. This study used a small sample size, and the Walls 2014 study may be seen as superseding this one; however, it is helpful to include this study for completeness, as the two studies pave the way for future research in this area. Because these are retrospective studies and some children don't receive the treatment for various reasons not related to research, there are no ethical dilemmas presented by gathering such data.

Baxter and Hughes (2018)

The published case series presented with photos in Chapter 15 shows speech and feeding improvements in all 5 children who had a release.[61] Many more cases of speech improvement are available. The authors propose a paradigm shift in the thinking regarding the condition of tongue-tie to encompass a "spectrum or continuum rather than a single disease state." All types of restrictions should be ruled out if the underlying symptoms and clinical history point to a tongue restriction being likely. The initial appearance may be misleading, as some fibers may be hidden beneath the surface and require further investigation. This case series is the first to link tongue-tie with speech delay in children. Two of the younger children (34 months old and 17 months old) had significant speech delays in addition to other speech difficulties and feeding issues. The older patient began using new words and combining words immediately after the release, which he had not previously done. The younger patient doubled her vocabulary the same day of the procedure, once her tongue was free, saying four new words: bubba, pawpaw, juice, and hot. Of note, she also stopped choking on liquids and spitting up, obviating the need for further medical testing to determine the cause of her swallowing difficulties. The article also highlights the importance of a team approach, with the tongue-tie release as an adjunct to speech therapy, not a replacement for therapy.

Tongue-tie "should be appreciated as a spectrum of restriction."[61]

The studies summarized above demonstrate that releasing a baby's tongue-tie can help that child develop normal speech in the future—and really, this concept is simple physics. If a person's mouth is sewn shut, he will likely have trouble speaking and eating. Similarly, if a surgeon goes in and stitches a person's tongue to the floor of his mouth, he will have trouble with speech (trying to talk with one's tongue held down can effectively simulate a tongue-tie!). How could it be controversial or surprising that after a tied-down tongue is released, speech and feeding improve? Unfortunately, a systematic review of this subject by Webb in 2013 claims that there is "no strong evidence that ankyloglossia causes speech problems."[69] Sadly, because of the lack of peer-reviewed journal articles in this field, the author concludes that there is no merit to the "common sense" argument that speech is impacted by a tethered tongue. Webb asserts that with the tongue-tip down rather than in the normal position of up, it is possible to articulate certain sounds, such as L or TH, but the abnormal tongue position causes the child to say the sound incorrectly and encourages him to compensate without realizing the effect on his speech. Articulation is only one measure of speech, and even though a child can say the L sound, it doesn't mean that during normal connected speech the child will say that sound correctly. I realized this fact firsthand when I once tried to ask for a sandwich with "light" sauce and received one with "white" sauce instead—because I was using the back of my mouth to produce the L sound that sounded like a W sound to my server. I still have to think about every L sound I make to say it correctly, and Apple's Siri still misunderstands some L sounds I make.

Tongue-tie release is an adjunct to speech therapy, not a replacement for therapy.

The research is lacking, but this in no way proves that speech is not impacted or that it does not improve after a tongue-tie release, either during infancy or childhood. It is only a matter of time until speech therapists, pediatricians, and other healthcare professionals see the difference a tongue-tie release can make to a child's speech. Children can quickly improve their speech once their tongues are free. The procedures are not magical and the improvements are not always immediate (although they can be), but tongue-tie releases can aid proper speech development. It is a medically necessary procedure that has the potential to drastically decrease therapy time and improve outcomes and quality of life for many children.

Section 4: More Issues

Many aspects of life are affected by a restricted tongue in addition to nursing, feeding, and speaking. Several of these bodily functions are vastly more important than the often-mentioned inability to lick an ice cream cone, play a wind instrument, or French kiss,[70-72] although those are important, too! Many seemingly unrelated issues such as enlarged tonsils and adenoids, multiple ear infections, sleep-disordered breathing, dental abnormalities, neck pain, and headaches can result from a tongue-tie. It's only relatively recently that the connections between these head and neck abnormalities and an underlying tongue-tie have become apparent, so research in these areas is just now being done. Understanding these connections can help parents and providers to recognize what to watch out for as these children develop, and earlier intervention should help prevent some of the dramatic corrective maxillofacial surgeries that these children sometimes require. In addition, the sequence of events, such as nursing problems, then feeding problems, then speech problems, along with neck pain, headaches, poor sleep, and crooked teeth requiring braces, can be halted before a child's (or adult's) quality of life is affected.

CHAPTER 19

Tonsils, Adenoids, and Tubes, Oh My!

Many children with tongue-ties also mouth breathe. Mouth breathing brings its own set of symptoms and is widely recognized as pathological. It leads to an open-mouth posture and changes in facial growth that can result in a long face pattern.[73,74] When the tongue does not rest on the roof of the mouth or palate as it should, an impaired swallow results and the palate is not expanded naturally. The palate grows into a V shape instead of a normal U shape; most often this is due to a tongue-tie.[75] The lowered position of the tongue also favors mouth breathing over nasal breathing.

When a young child's tongue-tie is released, the tongue automatically begins to rest up higher on the palate, and mouth breathing may resolve without additional therapy. The young child breathes through the nose, sleeps better and awakes feeling more rested. Older children and adults need retraining with a myofunctional therapist to learn to rest their tongue on the palate after years of bad habits and compensation. When the palate is not expanded, a child is much more likely to need braces and even extraction of permanent teeth (typically premolars) due to a lack of space in the underdeveloped upper jaw. When breastfeeding is difficult, and a bottle is used instead, the issue is compounded because the palate does not expand and flatten out from the natural action of nursing.[76] Many babies are born with high-arched palates from swallowing in utero with restricted tongues (beginning as early as 20 weeks), which are held to the floor of the mouth by tight lingual frena. Soft modern diets have a lot to do with causing narrow arches as well, but that concept is not part of the scope of this book (see *The Dental Diet* by Dr. Steven Lin for more).[77]

A tongue-tie prevents normal elevation of the middle and posterior portions of the tongue, and the result is a palate that is not normal. When pitted against each other, muscle vs. bone, the muscle always wins. The tongue is a powerful muscle and helps shape the palate and guide the growth of the bones in the oral cavity.[78] Once the teeth erupt, the tongue helps them to go into the proper alignment. The teeth rest in a neutral zone between the lips and the tongue. The resting force of the tongue alone provides enough force to contribute to malocclusion. Orthodontic forces that are very light move teeth and the accompanying bone. These habits that may appear benign in a young child may lead to unwanted dental bite changes, less than ideal oral functions, and facial changes. The upper jaw will be narrow and positioned not as far forward as normal, which happened to me. I had to have a palatal expander as a child, and then three sets of braces, culminating in jaw surgery that required my upper and lower jaws to be fractured and surgically repositioned. Is a tongue-tie the reason for all jaw discrepancies and jaw surgeries? Not likely. But without question it can contribute to poor tongue placement, mouth breathing, and unnatural jaw growth. Further, dysfunctional swallowing, oral habits, and other oral compensations can contribute to temporomandibular joint (TMJ) dysfunction and craniofacial pain syndromes that may begin during adolescence and continue into adulthood.

Mouth breathing can arise from various factors, but a tongue-tie should be considered as a potential and less identified cause. The nose is designed for breathing, and the mouth is designed for eating. Oral breathing leads to a host of issues, including oxygen deprivation, hyposmia or anosmia (poor or absent sense of smell), and nursing and feeding challenges for infants and older children. Mouth breathing can also put stress on a person and cause atypical functional muscle patterns, leading to poor growth of bones.[79] Oxygen is, without a doubt, the most critical nutrient our bodies need, and chronic oxygen deprivation can lead to chronic inflammation throughout the body.[80] Allergies and asthma also worsen in response to chronic mouth breathing.[81] Lastly, mouth breathing during the day and night has been linked to childhood eczema, or atopic dermatitis.[82]

A whole new field of dentistry is now focusing on treating both the airway and the "whole person" instead of simply the teeth. Airway orthodontics looks at crooked teeth from more than a cosmetic or dental viewpoint. These providers want to provide people with better-looking teeth while expanding the airway and allowing them to experience the benefits of proper muscle tone, airflow, and growth. They accomplish this by helping patients establish good habits such as nasal breathing and proper tongue and lip resting postures.[83]

Poor breathing can affect general health, but what does this have to do with tonsils, adenoids, and tubes? The palate is the floor of the nasal cavity. If the nasal cavity base is narrow due to a tongue-tie or high arched palate, the septum is likely to deviate, the airway will be smaller than normal, and the nasal airflow will be compromised. The airflow may become so difficult that the baby will begin to mouth breathe. This pattern of mouth breathing can continue throughout childhood and into adulthood. A caricature of a mouth breather is seen in the movie *Napoleon Dynamite*, where the main character has an elongated face, lip incompetence (his mouth won't close easily), and his mouth gapes open when he breathes. If an individual's nasal airflow is impaired and turbulent, it can cause microtrauma to the adenoids and tonsils, leading to increased inflammation of these tissues.[84] This trauma may cause them to enlarge, which starts a vicious cycle of airway obstruction leading to a worsening of the inflammation of the adenoids and tonsils until they obstruct the airway so significantly that removal is recommended. According to local otolaryngologists (ENTs), more children are having their tonsils removed for sleep reasons and mouth breathing than for infections these days. In fact, many children with undiagnosed tongue-ties have a history of having had their tonsils or adenoids removed. There are no published studies on the prevalence of children with a tongue-tie who have already had tonsils or adenoids removed at some point, but based on anecdotal and experiential evidence, it is very frequent.

When adenoids are enlarged, they can block the openings of the Eustachian tube into the throat. Children with tongue-ties also experience dysfunctional swallowing and impaired tongue mobility. This can be caused by a classic anterior tongue-tie or a posterior or hidden tongue-tie. When swallowing is impaired and the elevation of the tongue is limited, the Eustachian tube cannot open and equalize the pressure in the middle ear normally. The chief muscle that opens the tube, the tensor veli palatini, has difficulty doing so with an abnormal swallow.[85] When a person needs to equalize the pressure in the ears—for example, in a pressurized airplane or in a tall building's elevator—chewing bubblegum, yawning, or swallowing can open the Eustachian tube. Children with tongue-ties have difficulty with this and often suffer from chronic recurrent ear infections, leading to frequent consumption of antibiotics. Antimicrobials can negatively impact the gut microbiome and intestinal health, and increase antibiotic resistance in an individual or a population. Bottle-feeding may cause challenges for the Eustachian tubes as well. The tongue functions in an unnatural position when a foreign object like a bottle nipple is inserted in the mouth.[85] If the tongue is elevated and pushed back by the artificial nipple, it can block off the Eustachian tube.[85] Thumbsucking and pacifiers can promote the same tongue posture, and if the tongue is held down by a tongue-tie, the tongue often falls backward during sleep. When the tongue blocks the posterior pharynx, it can create varying degrees of airway obstruction and lead

> *When swallowing is impaired and the elevation of the tongue is limited, the Eustachian tube cannot open and equalize the pressure in the middle ear normally.*

to sleep-disordered breathing (see Chapter 20). The American Academy of Family Physicians and the American Academy of Pediatrics both recommend cessation of a pacifier around 6 to 10 months of age due to the increased risk of ear infections.[86]

Some children coming to evaluations for tongue-ties have had as many as 40 ear infections and 3 sets of ear tubes! Not all children with tongue-ties have ear infections, enlarged tonsils, and huge adenoids, but many do. Tonsillectomies, adenoidectomies, and myringotomies (ear tube placements) create physical, emotional, and financial strains on families. The recovery period after a tonsillectomy can be very uncomfortable for any age patient. All of these issues must be considered in the context of the unknown risks of general anesthesia to the developing brain. Therefore, it seems prudent to evaluate infants for tongue-ties at birth. It is possible that many developmental and functional abnormalities that lead to high healthcare costs could be prevented by a well-executed tongue-tie release.

CHAPTER 20

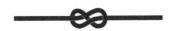

Sleep and Airway Issues

According to the Centers for Disease Control and Prevention, Americans are facing an epidemic of sleep issues. Thirty-five percent of adults state that they sleep 7 hours or less per night.[87] Many people have sleep apnea, hypopnea, or upper airway resistance syndrome, and even more snore. These varied disorders often have a lot to do with the anatomy and function of the upper airway. Snoring, which previously was thought to be merely annoying in adults and kids, and even cute in younger kids, is now a huge red flag indicating that something is likely wrong with that person's sleep. Bruxism or nighttime teeth grinding can also be related to sleep-disordered breathing and sleep apnea. It was once thought that tooth grinding was related to stress (and it certainly can be), but one likely reason children and adults grind their teeth at night may be because of airway obstruction. When a person goes to sleep and relaxes, and the airway is too small for any reason, the throat and mouth muscles will allow the tongue to obstruct the airway. Common reasons for a lack of space in the posterior pharynx are obesity and narrow airways (such as due to tongue-ties or a soft modern diet). When breathing is obstructed, the body tries to

If the tongue is held down by a tongue-tie, the tongue often falls backward during sleep and blocks the airway.

181

open the airway by protruding the mandible and grinding or clenching the teeth.[88,89] These actions are driven by low oxygen saturation.

Scientists now understand that, during sleep, the brain is hard at work consolidating memories and restoring itself. If a person wakes up often throughout the night due to the body's defense mechanism of arousing the person in order to force them to breathe, then that person will suffer from poor-quality sleep. When deciding whether to sleep or survive, the brainstem knows what needs to happen and wakes the person up. The problem is, if a person wakes up only partially, they do not realize that they have been awakened. Sometimes, these episodes, termed "micro-arousals," occur many times per hour, preventing the person from ever reaching the deep stages of sleep. Without a sleep study, you may not realize this pattern is even happening.

When breathing is obstructed, the body tries to open the airway by protruding the mandible and grinding or clenching the teeth.

In children, sleep-disordered breathing can lead to excessive daytime sleepiness and also symptoms that mimic attention deficit disorder (ADD) and attention deficit hyperactivity disorder (ADHD). According to one article, it is thought that 81% of children who snore and have ADD could have their symptoms eliminated by having their sleep issues treated.[90] In a more recent study, children ages 4 to 5 with ADHD were more likely than children without ADHD to have trouble sleeping due to enlarged adenoids. Older children ages 6 to 11 were more likely to have ADHD and sleep difficulty from enlarged tonsils because the adenoids tend to shrink by this age.[91] They also noted that the more severe the hypertrophy, the more severe the sleep trouble, and the more severe the ADHD symptoms.[91] The repeated hypoxia and low blood oxygen from sleep apnea affect brain function, and the repeated arousals do not allow restorative, restful sleep to occur. The researchers noted that the children with ADHD went to bed late, had a harder time falling asleep, had trouble staying asleep, and had more emotional and cognitive disorders from a lack of quality sleep.[91] Further, recent studies have shown that children with sleep apnea have reduced grey matter in the brain from delayed neuronal development or damaged neurons.[92,93] Children should undergo screening for sleep troubles at a minimum (there are several simple questionnaires that have been validated) and, ideally, undergo sleep studies before being placed on medications for ADD. Quality sleep is much more important than we previously realized.

What does a tongue-tie have to do with sleep? As we've seen previously, the tongue-tie and low tongue resting posture can lead to mouth breathing. Mouth breathing prevents the brain from experiencing the deepest levels of sleep; therefore, people who mouth breathe awaken unrefreshed by their recent sleep. Children and adults may get the right quantity of sleep at night, but many are not getting the right quality of sleep they need. Snoring from upper airway resistance can be a warning sign of obstructive sleep apnea or sleep-disordered breathing. The tongue-tie release in infancy combined with nursing can prevent this phenomenon by helping the infant develop a broad, flat palate and well-developed nasal passages and sinuses. A tongue-tied baby's oral cavity does not grow and develop optimally.[3] The jaws are small, and the tongue is pushed backward into the throat. The tongue should rest up in the palate and help to expand the palate. If the palate is narrow and the lower jaw is restricted or retruded, the lower jaw also takes up airway space. Held back, the only place left for the tongue to go is backward, which closes off part of the airway. A narrow palate and soft palate elongation have been associated with tongue-ties in a recent study.[64] After full tongue-tie releases, children are consistently found to sleep more deeply, snore less, exhibit fewer movements, and feel more refreshed in the morning.

> *Children and adults may get the right quantity of sleep at night, but many are not getting the right quality of sleep they need.*

Often they concentrate better and are less hyperactive as well. It is fascinating that a tiny string can have such a dramatic impact on human physiology and quality of life.

A narrow palate leads to a decrease in airway volume in the nasal cavity, and with a reduction in airway volume, the airflow resistance is increased by the fourth power. In other words, an airway half as small is 16 times harder for air to flow through when breathing. The good news is that a process as simple as an orthodontic palatal expander can increase the nasal cavity volume, and it appears that the change is permanent. It decreases airway resistance and makes it easier for the child to breathe nasally.[94] Tonsillectomy and adenoidectomy in combination with maxillary expansion seem to aid in reducing obstructive sleep apnea and sleep-disordered breathing. The benefits of the three procedures are additive. The order in which the procedures are performed does not seem to matter as much as the fact that both expansion and reduction of lymphoid tissue are performed.[95]

Sometimes a combination of tongue-tie release and maxillary expansion (a palatal expander) or growth appliance can benefit the child as well, although research on this modality to reduce obstructive sleep apnea or sleep-disordered breathing is lacking. Anecdotal and experiential evidence, however, suggests that this method works, too. Releasing the tongue and expanding the palate allow the tongue to move out of the airway and rest up in the palate, and also increase nasal volume (thereby decreasing airflow resistance) so the child can breathe through the nose. Nasal breathing can reduce the microtrauma to the tonsils and adenoids that mouth breathing causes, which may shrink the tonsils and adenoids, and in some cases eliminate the need for surgery.

Bedwetting is a common finding in children and is difficult to manage. Often bedwetting occurs due to a lack of deep sleep. Children (and adults) with sleep-disordered breathing have frequent arousals or micro-arousals, which can cause the child to have the urge to urinate. Sleep-disordered breathing has been associated with nighttime bed wetting, and a recent systematic review of removing tonsils and adenoids showed that bedwetting improved in more than 60% of the patients and 50% had a complete resolution of symptoms.[96] In many patients suffering from bedwetting, a simple tongue-tie release (which carries less morbidity than tonsillectomy) can allow the child to achieve deeper sleep levels and stop bedwetting—sometimes even the same night. The removal of tonsils and adenoids, the application of a maxillary expander, and the performance of a tongue-tie release can all work together to improve sleep quality and quantity.

CHAPTER 21

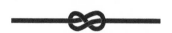

Dental Issues

Tongue- and lip-ties can cause dental issues in toddlers, children of all ages, and even adults. The problems may include gum recession, difficult-to-clean areas, crooked teeth, or malocclusions. As discussed earlier, sometimes seemingly insignificant issues like tooth grinding, or bruxism, can be a sign of deeper issues, such as sleep disturbances and airway compromise. The U.S. Surgeon General famously made the public aware that the mouth is a "mirror of general health and well-being" and highlighted the important role that dental health can play in the health of the rest of the body.[97] As research and clinical knowledge increase, this statement is becoming more fully validated than ever before. This book discusses an example of this principle, in that there are many seemingly unrelated issues that are affected by this "tiny string under the tongue."

Lip-Ties and Diastemas (Gap in the Teeth)

The first and most obvious dental issue related to a tethered oral tissue, in this case a lip-tie, is a diastema, which is a gap between the front teeth. A lip-tie can cause a gap between the top teeth, and a tongue-tie can cause a gap between the bottom teeth (incisors). The tendency to grow a gap between the front teeth is often hereditary, passed down from generation to generation as a dominant gene, because the same process that leads to a lip-tie also often leads to a diastema.

A thick, restrictive lip-tie can also cause food or milk to become trapped in the pocket between the lip and the teeth, leading to dental decay in infants to adolescents.[53] Initially, decay will start as a white line on the tooth near the gum line and then turn into a white patch, until finally the enamel is so soft from losing calcium that the surface breaks and leaves a hole, or cavity. This presentation occurs very frequently among dental patients whose parents don't realize their child has a lip-tie. A lip-tie can cause pain when the upper front teeth are brushed (most often in toddlers) and the toothbrush hits the frenum. When a parent lifts the lip to assist with brushing, the tightness of the attachment can also hurt the child. Either way, it is harder for the parent to brush the child's teeth, which, along with food becoming trapped next to the front teeth, can certainly put a child at risk for dental caries.

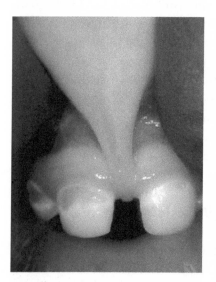 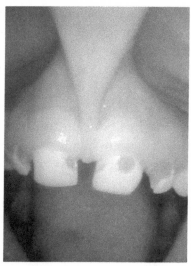

A lip-tie causes difficulty brushing and traps food or liquid by the teeth, thus putting the child at risk for cavities.

In some cases, a healthcare provider will tell parents not to worry about a maxillary lip-tie because children often fall down and rip the frenum, effectively giving themselves a frenectomy. While this advice sounds helpful at first, if this does happen, it bleeds significantly, causes distress to parent and child, and does not actually remove the tissue between the teeth, resulting in an incomplete release. Unfortunately, this advice also extends to tongue-ties, with the myth that the child can fall down and rip the tongue-tie as well (or they advise it will stretch). It is virtually impossible to rip a tongue-tie from a fall, because it is hidden behind the teeth, and advising parents to treat either medical condition by future trauma is unhelpful at best.

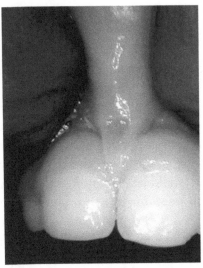

Incomplete release from a fall, which resulted in significant bleeding. Notice the tissue is still attached and will heal back together within a few weeks.

If a child has cavities at age 2 or 3 years, it can be difficult to treat them. And depending on the size and number of cavities present, the child will likely need sedation or general anesthesia to make it possible for the dentist to be able to restore the teeth. Thus, it is best to release the lip-tie if it is making it difficult to brush, or the parent is having to fight with the child nightly to brush that particular area. Using scissors to release a lip-tie fully is nearly impossible because of the thickness of the scissors blades and the thickness of the gingiva. A simple snip will alleviate some tension but will leave a fleshy piece of the lip still embedded in the gums and will not typically allow for gap closure. By contrast, using a laser for the release allows the surgeon to remove the entire attachment in a matter of seconds, with little to no bleeding and minimal discomfort. There really is no contest between the available methods for releasing a lip-tie; the newer laser technology has no rival.

Many children have a gap between their front teeth. Should every frenum receive treatment with a laser? No. Interdental spacing between primary teeth is actually normal, and as long as it is evenly distributed, it is a good thing, because it is an indicator of sufficient space for the permanent teeth to erupt with minimal crowding. Even a gap solely between the two front teeth does not automatically require treatment. A functional evaluation by a trained tongue-tie release provider is helpful. If the gap is sufficiently large (larger than a few millimeters), there may be a reason to release it. If it is causing the child to have difficulty brushing the upper teeth or if food is getting trapped under the lip, and there's a wide gap, the benefits likely outweigh the risks in favor of doing the laser procedure. It would be extraordinarily rare that a child would need to be put to sleep for this procedure, or have it performed with scissors. With a skilled provider and a high-quality laser, it is easily accomplished in about 20 seconds in the office setting, with minimal discomfort and distress to the child. Typically, if the child is younger than 18 months old and the canines have not erupted, the gap will close significantly, if not totally, in a matter of weeks to months after a release. If the child is older than 18 months old but the tie is still causing functional issues, such as difficulty eating from a spoon or producing speech sounds, the lip can be released at any age. The next best time to release the upper lip for gap closure seems to be when the permanent teeth are just starting to erupt or have just come into the mouth.[17] There is a normal movement of the teeth at this stage, and once all the permanent teeth are in, there is much less normal migration of teeth that could help close the gap without braces. This procedure could limit the need for braces (at least for the reason of a diastema), but it is certainly not a guarantee. In an older child, releasing the lip with a laser is a simple procedure that causes minimal discomfort, which can easily be controlled with ibuprofen or acetaminophen.

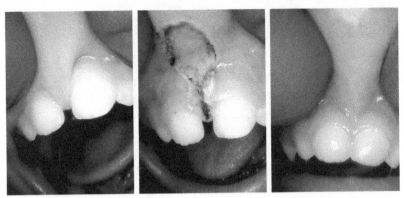

Significant gap closure when released before primary canines erupt.

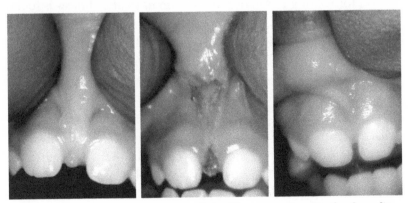

Significantly easier oral hygiene and significant gap closure after laser lip-tie release.

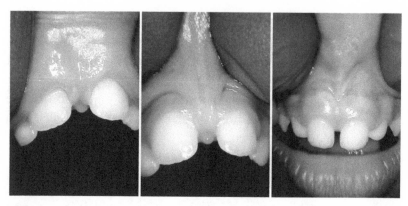

Thick frenum causing difficulty brushing teeth (left), blanching of frenum (middle), and six months after release (right). The patient had improved lip mobility, easier brushing, significant gap closure, and no scarring. The rest of the gap should close when permanent teeth erupt.

Some dentists may prefer that parents wait until after a child's braces are removed before having a provider release the frenum. This is an outdated recommendation based on a suggestion from an orthodontist at the beginning of the 20th century. The most cited reason for waiting to remove the frenum until after braces is found in Bishara (1972), in which he echoes the opinion that "it seems preferable to close the spaces orthodontically as early as possible during treatment and then to perform the surgical procedure."[98] This recommendation, however, is solely the opinion of that provider and is not based on evidence. The concern was that the release of the frenum could cause scar tissue to form and interfere with the teeth closing together. Since that time, it has been observed that after a frenectomy, the teeth come together in a matter of weeks to months on their own with no orthodontic intervention. Recently, Dr. Kotlow was able to have this unhelpful recommendation—to wait until permanent teeth erupt to release the lip-tie—removed from the treatment guidelines of the American Academy of Pediatric Dentistry, which are evidence-based. Some people also worry that the release will give the child a "gummy smile," but there is no reason to think that releasing the lip-tie will cause a gummy smile in a patient who would not have had one otherwise. Releasing the lip does not often change the child's normal lip resting position or smiling lip resting position. Instead, it gives them a greater chance at normal mobility and function, and it often allows for closure of the gap without the need for braces.

The gap between the upper teeth will often close on its own if it is 2 mm wide or smaller. In these cases, parents may wait to release the ties if there are no other functional issues or difficulty with oral hygiene. Such ties can be reassessed and released when the children are older and the permanent incisors are erupting, which is between ages 7 and 9, if the procedure is needed. Often the procedure is not needed in this group of patients, and parents are advised to wait and see how the children grow. Each case should be handled individually, and the best research and clinical judgment available at the time should be used to determine what is best for each child.

> *The best time to perform the procedure for gap closure is before 18 months old or when the permanent teeth are erupting.*
> *- Larry Kotlow, DDS*[17]

Tooth Grinding (Bruxism)

Tooth grinding was previously thought to be related to stress in a child or parent's life. The more stress, the more grinding. Certainly, this can be true, and grinding may sometimes be a result of increased stress. However, nighttime grinding of the teeth, or bruxism, can be a warning sign of something else. The new thinking is that nighttime teeth grinding (which sounds like nails on a chalkboard to many parents!) can actually be a sign of sleep-disordered breathing, which was discussed in the previous chapter. This could be related to a tongue-tie, because the tongue-tie holds the base of the tongue down instead of allowing it to assume its normal resting position on the palate. As the muscles of the body relax during sleep, the tongue can fall backward and obstruct the airway, causing difficulty breathing. It is hypothesized that the brain then causes the teeth to grind in an effort to arouse the child (or adult) to a lighter state of sleep—and also protrude the lower jaw to facilitate an open airway and easier breathing.

Bruxism is often a warning sign of something else.

Gum Recession

Gum recession is a common finding in a patient with a tongue-tie, but can also occur from lip and buccal ties. The strong muscles of the tongue, lips, or cheeks will pull on the gums over time and exert a traumatic force that will cause the gum tissues to slowly pull away from the teeth, leaving exposed roots. Recession is commonly found on the insides of the lower incisors from tongue-ties, the outsides of the lower incisors or outsides of the upper incisors from lip-ties, or on the canines or premolars from buccal ties. Once the frena are removed and the traumatic forces are mitigated, the tissues will sometimes rebound and lessen the recession, but often the defects will remain. The recession should halt and not get any worse if gentle tooth brushing is practiced. It is important for the patient to do stretching exercises to keep the tissues separated and prevent the frenum wound from re-forming a tight attachment. A gum graft may be necessary, but often a graft can be avoided if a tight frenum is removed when recession is first observed.

Cavities (Dental Caries)

Dental caries are often seen with greater prevalence in children and adults with tongue-ties or lip-ties. As discussed earlier, the lip can trap food next to the teeth and make it difficult to brush them. The tongue performs many functions, but one of its main functions in addition to forming boluses to swallow is cleaning up the remaining food particles and swallowing them, too. Sometimes a child (or adult) will have a tongue-tie and find that food becomes stuck between the cheeks and teeth because the tongue is so restricted it cannot clean the back teeth. Often these patients must stick their fingers in their mouths in order to clean food debris from the teeth because their tongues are not able to do so properly; this is known as oral toilet. One of the first things people notice when they have their tongue-ties released is that their tongues can now touch the back teeth and clean them for the first time! Food can also become stuck on the palate and cause people to have to use their fingers to free it. These habits can be quite off-putting when people are eating in public.

Braces and Jaw Surgery

Braces or orthodontics are frequently required in patients with tongue-ties or lip-ties. As already discussed, a restrictive frenum can create a gap between the teeth that requires braces, but additional problems can arise from tight pieces of tissue that restrict growth. One or both jaw bones can be affected by a tongue-tie, which can cause the bones to grow too little, set up dental crowding issues, prevent the jaws from fitting together properly, and ultimately require jaw surgery. Sadly, I experienced this aspect of tongue-tie myself. I had an undiagnosed tongue-tie, so my tongue rested on the floor of the mouth instead of on my palate. This resting position inhibited the growth of my upper jaw, or maxilla. I needed braces and an expander around the age of seven, braces again from 11 to 13, and finally, very complex and expensive maxillofacial surgery with braces a third time as I was graduating from high school and starting college.

Jaw surgery is only performed once the jaws stop growing, normally around age 16 in girls or age 18 in boys. Young adults experience many emotional and physical changes during the teenage years, and extensive surgery and braces can present a significant psychosocial challenge to them. In addition to jaw-related problems, the temporomandibular joint (TMJ) can be affected as well, and it was in my case. I developed degenerative changes in the disks by age 18, so during the jaw surgery they also operated on those joints, and I have had stiffness in the joints ever since. All of these sequelae can and do arise from tongue-ties. If these issues could be prevented by tongue-ties being diagnosed and addressed at birth, significant healthcare costs and morbidity could be avoided. Even if tethered oral tissues are not released until early childhood, the necessity for braces and subsequent jaw surgery should dramatically decrease. The benefits of the releases are enhanced when they are combined with myofunctional therapy, which helps to re-establish proper balance between orofacial musculature and the resting posture of the tongue. A tongue-tie release combined with myofunctional therapy can help prevent relapse in orthodontic cases (needing braces again) and can also be beneficial in surgical orthodontic cases.

Orthodontics, or braces, are systems of oral appliances and brackets used to apply sustained forces in specific areas of the teeth and jaws to move teeth over time. They are needed when there are imbalances between the forces of the tongue, lips, and cheeks as well as growth discrepancies in the jaw bones that lead to too little room for the teeth, or dental crowding. Most children with tongue-ties are born with high-arched palates at birth. This is not good for the teeth or the airway. Because the palate is the floor of the nasal cavity, these children are more likely to have deviated nasal septa, narrowed airways, impaired sinuses, and increased nasal airway resistance, leading to increased mouth breathing, which exacerbates their problems.

A high-arched palate in a baby will often flatten out to a more normal U shape from a V shape with tongue-tie release and proper nursing. Bottle-feeding does not offer the same advantages, as Dr. Brian Palmer's work shows.[76] A V-shaped palate does not allow enough arch circumference to accommodate all of the teeth, and therefore they erupt misaligned, on top of each other, or there's not enough room to erupt at all (impacted teeth like canines or wisdom teeth). Children with very little room and extensive crowding often need premolar (bicuspid) teeth extracted. These extractions can make the airway problem worse and lead to more issues with breathing down the road. It is better to try to avoid extracting permanent teeth because a smaller arch leads to breathing issues, which lead to less oxygen in the body, and that has far-reaching effects more significant than just straight teeth. Expansion and growth appliances are a better idea than extracting and retracting the teeth in the majority of cases. Most of those who need palatal expanders have tongue-ties. Most people who need jaw surgery also likely have tongue-ties. Orthodontic interventions are one of the most expensive costs of raising a child, and many families cannot afford braces, which are considered a luxury when compared to food, clothing and shelter. When viewed from the perspective of preventing future morbidity and expensive corrective procedures like orthodontia and jaw surgery, the tongue-tie release can be seen for what it is: an enormously cost-effective, life-enhancing gift.

CHAPTER 22

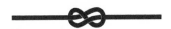

Additional Associations with Tongue-Tie

Little formalized research exists related to this next discussion, so the reader is encouraged to make his or her own observations and consider contributing to the pool of meaning in this area. The associations that follow are so new that there hasn't been time to study them or to tease the tongue-tie piece from the greater disease process. One day these observations may be better understood, but for now, it is interesting to look for connections between different conditions by compiling the many stories of patients who have seen relief from them.

Midline field defects, or simply midline defects, are a collection of congenital conditions that occur in the midline of the body. Examples include cleft lips and palates, congenital heart malformations, spina bifida, sacral dimples, hypospadias, imperforate ani, and omphaloceles, to name a few.[99] Tongue-ties and lip-ties are also considered midline defects. These congenital conditions and more have been associated tongue- and lip-ties. Does every child with a tongue-tie have these issues? Certainly not. Do some children with these issues also have a tongue or lip-tie? Perhaps, which is why they should be evaluated by trained professionals who have experience with tethered oral tissues. Not every boy with hypospadias (a condition in which the urethra does not come out of its usual location on the penis) has a tongue-tie, but many have seen the connection, so these babies should be checked. The same goes for infants with cleft palates, sacral dimples, and congenital heart problems.

There is an enzyme called methylenetetrahydrofolate reductase, but it is commonly referred to by its abbreviation: MTHFR. This enzyme deals with methylation, or the way the body processes toxins and repairs DNA. Variations and mutations in the gene encoding the enzyme have been associated with midline defects and also with tongue-ties. This association is not definitive, and not everyone with MTHFR has a tongue-tie. It is a complex interaction but worth mentioning. Methylation and MTHFR are involved in DNA expression and epigenetics, an emerging and fascinating field of medicine. Even though your DNA says one thing, whether that gene is turned on, to what extent it is turned on, and when it is turned on, are related to epigenetics, or factors outside of your DNA. You can send a saliva sample to a DNA processing company that will sequence the DNA, which can be uploaded to a third-party website to tell you your MTHFR variants.

The two common MTHFR gene variants are A1298C and C677T, but in some countries, up to 50% of the population has a variation from normal in one of these locations in the DNA. This variation can lead to reduced activity in MTHFR and reduced methylation. Some experts believe that mothers who have a variant in MTHFR should supplement with an active form of folate instead of folic acid, which, since 1992 in the United States, has been recommended for all pregnant women to reduce the risk of neural tube birth defects such as spina bifida. Folic acid is a synthetic form of folate that must undergo several reactions in the body to become a usable form of folate. However, folic acid is also added to grains such as bread, cereals, and other processed foods, so a large amount of folic acid is being consumed by the public, and especially pregnant women.

A person with reduced MTHFR activity has difficulty changing folic acid into the form the body needs, folate, and this extra folic acid can prevent the body from using folate, potentially creating a deficiency by having so much of the inactive form of folic acid floating around the bloodstream. So a better way to supplement (instead of folic acid) may be the active form (folate, L-5-methylfolate, or L-5-MTHF), which does not require an extra step to be activated.

In a few studies, folic acid supplementation has been shown to increase cancer rates[100] and speed up tumor growth,[101] and it can also mask a vitamin B12 deficiency.[102] Many of the studies on MTHFR and heart defects, Down syndrome, and ADHD, for example, are inconclusive, and some are conflicting.[103] The connection between MTHFR and myelomeningocele and spina bifida is greater, but not definitive. Because MTHFR, folate, and methylation are intricately involved in both neural crest closure and programmed cell death (apoptosis), it makes sense that tongue-tie, which involves migration of cells and failure of apoptosis of neuroectoderm, would be related to folate, methylation, and MTHFR. One article mentions a relative folate deficiency at the cellular level as a cause for neural tube defects,[104] which could also be caused by an oversupply of folic acid blocking the active form of folate from reaching its target. Most likely, MTHFR is just the tip of the iceberg, and the actual mechanism of increasing tongue-tie prevalence in the population is complex. As with most conditions, it is not a simple case of "this gene causes tongue-tie," or it would have been found by now.

It is not a simple case of "this gene causes tongue-tie," or it would have been found by now.

Why is tongue-tie prevalence increasing?

Tongue-tie diagnosis appears to be on the rise, and this is due to many factors. Primarily, it may be attributed to the rise in breastfeeding initiation rates and the discovery of nursing issues for mom and baby, as well as an increase in tongue-tie awareness. There is a renewed interest in treating tongue-tie, and technological advances and the ease in which the tongue is released by laser have facilitated a much easier route to correction. If a mother were to choose between general anesthesia to correct a tongue-tie and switching to formula, many would choose formula. For many moms, the incomplete scissors clip or snip did not solve the problem, and that's why the laser option has gained such popularity. If the choice is between a rapid in-office laser procedure or abandoning breastfeeding, many are now choosing to proceed with the procedure (not to mention the other health benefits discussed throughout the book). Also, just switching to bottles or formula doesn't magically correct the tongue-tie. Those babies (and their families) still struggle with feeding issues, and they can suffer from horrible gas pains, colic, and reflux, along with choking and gagging while eating.

Seasoned practitioners might say that treating tongue-tie is a "fad," but I would argue that treating tongue-tie is no more of a fad than treating autism. According to the Centers for Disease Control and Prevention, the diagnosis of autism has risen from 1 in 150 children in the year 2000 to 1 in 59 children today,[105] and that rise is largely due to increased awareness of the condition and its signs, symptoms, and functional impacts on quality of life, as well as an increasing number of children affected. The diagnosis of tongue-tie is similar, and it is likely due to a combination of increased awareness and increased prevalence. Tongue-tie can certainly be hereditary. In many families, when one child has struggles, typically with nursing, the parents realize one or many of the older children have symptoms of a tongue-tie; upon examination, their suspicions are generally confirmed. Often when a baby or child is identified with a tongue-tie, one or both parents realize they also have functional issues and symptoms of a tie. Upon examination, they also learn they have a restriction (and, when the tie is released, a resolution of symptoms as well, indicating that was the cause of their issues). Tongue-ties are partly increasing due to decades of unrecognized tongue-ties and the influence of a dominant gene on a population. One parent can pass it on to all or most of his or her children, creating a compounding effect. However, another piece of the puzzle likely includes our modern environment and diet causing epigenetic changes (our environment affecting genetic expression). We're seeing new and greater problems, potentially from our exposure to environmental factors such as increased ultrasound in utero, increased time indoors, chemicals such as glyphosate (Roundup®), toxins, flame retardants, and processed or genetically modified foods introduced into our bodies, leading to increasing cases of autism, diabetes, cancer, autoimmune issues, and also tongue-tie. But again, scientists are just now learning all the effects our modern environment is having on our bodies, and further research is needed.

The diagnosis of tongue-tie is similar, and it is likely due to a combination of increased awareness and increased prevalence.

The Social and Psychological Impact of Tethered Tissues

The seemingly inconsequential issues arising from a tongue-tie can cause surprisingly wide-reaching problems, including psychological and interpersonal issues. One child we saw in our office had the thickest to-the-tip tongue-tie that I had ever seen. He had cavities on many teeth, muffled speech and would hardly talk, and was very shy. I imagine that every time he spoke, someone had to ask him, "What did you say?" or clearly couldn't understand him, so he would just turn inward and shut down. In fact, after we released his tongue-tie, we saw his brother a couple of months later for his routine cleaning. His brother reported that he is like a different kid! He is now talkative and more outgoing, and he speaks more clearly.

A child who had a speech impediment her whole life struggled to be understood by her friends on her softball team. A girl's social interactions during her formative years can truly alter the way she thinks about herself for a lifetime. Her father remarked a month after her release that her softball coaches were noticing that she seemed happier and was interacting with the other children more. He also noted that children were no longer always asking the adults

203

around her, "What did she say?" He said, "it is no understatement to say that releasing her tongue has changed her life."

Recently, a grandmother told of a boy in her class over 60 years ago who was tongue-tied. She said the teachers would have him speak in front of the class to try and make him talk more and get over his shyness; sadly, both the teachers and the other students were mean to him. Although he was bright, he was ridiculed and ostracized because the children knew he couldn't speak well. When he was a teenager, he committed suicide, the grandmother said, because he had been so mistreated and rejected due to the speech difficulties resulting from the tongue-tie. The psychological impact on tongue-tied children and adults has been greatly minimized, and the often-seen social benefits of the release (and the possible detrimental effect of inaction) should be discussed with patients and their parents.

Children are blamed for all kinds of feeding issues (picky eating, eating slowly, smacking, or eating with their mouth open), speech issues (mumbling and so-called baby talk), and for being shy in order to hide their eating and speech troubles. Even psychological issues such as depression, ADD, ADHD, and bedwetting can be related to tongue-ties, as we've seen. These issues don't even include the psychological issues related to nursing for mothers, which can include feeling like a failure for something that should, in their minds, come naturally, and postpartum depression or post-traumatic stress disorder (PTSD) from being repeatedly hurt by one's baby while nursing (and feeling guilty for feeling that way). Often during the visit in our office, the mother will break down and begin to cry as she describes how difficult it has been and how frustrated she is that none of her healthcare providers have identified this condition, and how much pain and suffering both she and the baby have been through. Certainly, there are hormones at play, but these mothers have been through war, battling every day and struggling for weeks and months to feed their babies. The psychological impact of a tongue-tie on patients and their families should be investigated by the prudent practitioner and treated with therapy if indicated. For primary care providers and others to say there is "nothing wrong" or "everything's fine" because the baby is gaining weight, despite all these other issues (which are ignored or brushed off), is, frankly, malpractice.

Neck Tension and Pain

In adults and even children, a restrictive tongue pulls the hyoid bone in the neck upward and puts tension on all of the connective tissue or fascia in the neck, which is connected throughout the whole body. Neck tension, pain, and range of motion often improve significantly after a tongue-tie release, and this is corroborated by physical therapists and chiropractors who have seen the patient weekly, sometimes for years, and are shocked by the difference. Often when we release an adult, they will report that they no longer have to (and, in fact, do not have the ability to) pop their knuckles or pop their neck to release tension in the connective tissue. Is there any evidence in the scientific literature of tongue-tie release helping to alleviate popping knuckles? No, because no one would spend money to investigate popping knuckles. However, we have seen the results often in our office, and others across the country have observed this as well. At the same time, these people will often report feeling less anxiety and as if a weight has been lifted when their tongue is released. The constant tension in the neck radiates throughout the body and puts the person in an unrealized state of stress and fight-or-flight response of the sympathetic nervous system. This extra adrenaline and sympathetic response can also create digestive issues, such as irritable bowel syndrome, which is difficult to treat, leads to headaches, and a feeling of anxiety and even depression. Releasing this tiny string can have profound impacts on an individual's daily life.

Do all patients suffering from tongue-tie have these symptoms? Certainly not, and the presentation is variable. Some people have speech and feeding issues, whereas others have dental issues, migraines, and anxiety, and others have any number of combinations of symptoms. Will release take away all of the symptoms? Often it will help many, but not all of the symptoms, but sometimes it alleviates problems that an individual didn't even realize were affecting them, such as poor sleep. The procedure is so low risk, and the soreness lasts for just a few days, that if releasing the tie could potentially help that patient at all, the rewards far outweighs the risks.

CHAPTER 23

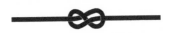

Myofunctional Therapy

Paula Fabbie, RDH, BS, COM and
Lorraine Frey RDH, LDH, BAS, COM, FAADH

The following chapter is an excerpt from the authors' soon-to-be-released publication,
The Miracle of Orofacial Myofunctional Therapy: A Parent's Must-Have Guide
for Information, Resources, and Easy to Implement Strategies.

You may wonder why you've never heard of orofacial myofunctional therapy. That is mainly because the public still remains largely uninformed that this amazing therapy exists. Currently, there is a shortage of well-educated healthcare professionals who are knowledgeable about orofacial myofunctional disorders (OMDs) and how these disorders can affect sleep, breathing, chewing, swallowing, growth and development, behavior, school performance, and some speech issues. Additionally, there is a shortage of qualified and experienced therapists, and we encourage those professionals who are qualified to pursue the necessary education and training opportunities to meet this growing need.

Healthcare professionals and parents alike are becoming more interested in holistically focused solutions to these problems. Currently, however, there are very few professional schools that offer the basics regarding identification and treatment of these disorders, yet the demand for this therapy is increasing.

Experts agree that early treatment produces the best and least expensive results. Parents are hungry for this information and, at times, express frustration and disappointment that their child's OMDs weren't addressed early enough. Our goal is to help parents recognize OMDs, learn when to seek help, provide resources, and enable parents to be in a position to make well-informed decisions regarding their child's health.

The History of Myofunctional Therapy: How did myofunctional therapy evolve?

Orofacial myofunctional therapy, or OMT as it is commonly referred to, dates back to the early 1900s. One prominent article, "Exercises for the Development of the Muscles of the Face, with View to Increasing Their Functional Activity," was published in 1918.[106] The author, Alfred Paul Rodgers, DDS, described myofunctional therapy and proper tongue positioning in the oral cavity to improve jaw growth, nasal breathing, and facial appearance.

In the 1960s, OMT exercises were pioneered by orthodontist Walter Straub to assist in reeducating an atypical swallow. From the 1960s to present day, interest in orofacial myofunctional therapy has increased significantly. Why now? Evidence-based research by pediatric sleep experts conclude that OMT is a viable treatment option and they are advocating for and driving this resurgence.

In a large multi-year study completed in 2012, epidemiologist Karen Bonuck, PhD, concluded that in children ages 6 months to 7 years, snoring, obstructive sleep apnea, and mouth breathing contribute to neurobehavior morbidity, including greatly increased risk of ADHD, peer-to-peer behavior problems, and increased aggression and anxiety.[107]

Writing in the journal *Sleep*, Stanford researchers Camacho et al. (2015) concluded after a systematic review that OMT improves sleep apnea by approximately 50% in adults and 62% in children. The researchers also determined that myofunctional therapy could serve to assist with other OSA treatments as well.[108]

Dentists and orthodontists are aware of the harm caused by orofacial myofunctional disorders. These disorders include thumb, finger, and object sucking, nail biting, lip licking and biting, tongue thrust, jaw thrusting, excessive drooling, sloppy eating and open mouth chewing, improper swallowing, food/texture aversions, clenching and grinding the teeth, and mouth breathing.

New evidence suggests that there is so much more involved with tongue thrust, non-nutritive sucking, and poor rest postures. Pediatric sleep experts are looking at improper facial and jaw growth, which has an impact on the upper airway. These improper rest postures and noxious habits may play a role in the development of sleep-disordered breathing and obstructive sleep apnea. The presence of snoring in a child should be addressed, according to Pediatric Clinical Guidelines. Family history of obstructive sleep apnea (OSA) and disruptive snoring is commonly found among children who exhibit these symptoms."[109]

According to the authors of the text *Contemporary Orthodontics*, "Because of rapid growth exhibited by children during the primary dentition years, it would seem that treatment of jaw discrepancies by growth modification should be successful at a very early age. If treated from ages 4 to 6 when rapid growth occurs, significant improvements in skeletal discrepancies can be accomplished in a short period of time." The authors, Proffitt et al. (2006), concluded that "stability of these results are dependent on eliminated OMDs and establishing harmonious muscle function."[110]

During a comprehensive evaluation, an orofacial myofunctional therapist will use various techniques to assess function, take measurements, and make observations after collecting a thorough medical, dental, and sleep history. Orofacial myofunctional therapy does not involve invasive procedures and is not a manipulative therapy.

Orofacial Myofunctional Therapy: What Every Parent NEEDS to Know

Symptoms of Orofacial Myofunctional Disorders

Does your child suffer or struggle with...
- » Congestion/mouth breathing
- » Open mouth posture at rest
- » Allergies
- » Low tone
- » Dental crowding/crossbite/open bite
- » High and narrow palate
- » Tongue-tie
- » Drooling
- » Dark circles under the eyes
- » Thumb or object sucking
- » Nail biting
- » Bedwetting
- » Open mouth chewing/sloppy eating

What are the signs of orofacial myofunctional disorders (OMDs)?

The Nose
- » Nasal congestion that encourages mouth breathing
- » Loud audible breathing
- » Overbreathing/hyperventilation
- » Excessive yawning
- » Sniffling
- » Frequent sighs
- » Visible movements of upper chest/shoulders when breathing

The Lips

- » Open mouth posture—lips that are parted most of the time
- » Dry, chapped, cracked lips
- » Flaccid, low tone
- » Large, rolled lower lip
- » Lip licking
- » Lip biting
- » Lip sucking
- » Visible saliva at corners of mouth
- » Excessive drooling and inability to control saliva

The Tongue

- » Visible at rest
- » Visible during speech
- » Tongue thrust
- » Appears large and in the way
- » Scalloped edges
- » Tongue-tie

The Mandible (the lower jaw)

- » Jaw tendency to shift left, right, or forward
- » Jaws that don't fit together
- » Headaches/facial pain
- » Jaws that appear to be mismatched
- » Clicking, popping, or noise
- » Ear ringing
- » Unable to open wide
- » Sudden change in the bite
- » Excessive gum chewing
- » Excessive leaning on the hands to support posture

Daytime Breathing
  » Audible breathing
  » Predominant mouth breathing during speech, eating, and daily activities or
  » when concentrating
  » Large tonsils and adenoids that block the airway

Sleep
  » Snoring
  » Noisy breathing
  » Grinding or clenching of the teeth
  » Witnessed apnea (when the child stops breathing)
  » Sweating
  » Recurring nightmares
  » Bedwetting
  » Restless sleep or excessive movement
  » Open mouth posture
  » Hyperextended neck posture
  » Difficulty waking up in the morning
  » Daytime sleepiness or irritability
  » Moodiness and behavior issues
  » Hyperactivity and cognitive problems

Habits
  » Thumbsucking/digit sucking/object sucking
  » Nail biting/cuticle biting
  » Hands or objects in mouth
  » Lip licking, lip sucking, lip biting
  » Tendency to chew on everything
  » Mouth breathing
  » Nose picking
  » Skin picking, hair pulling
  » Eyebrow/eyelash picking
  » Skin biting
  » Frequent throat clearing

- » Coughing in the absence of illness
- » Jaw popping
- » Neck adjusting
- » Knuckle cracking
- » Blanket sucking
- » Excessive Gum chewing

With this knowledge, we encourage parents to address the above-mentioned symptoms early and appropriately, under the guidance of experienced and properly trained clinicians.

What is orofacial myofunctional therapy?

Orofacial myofunctional therapy involves proper tongue positioning to improve oral and facial muscle function and tone, promote nasal breathing, and improve craniofacial and oral rest postures. Due to current research and many studies conducted by Stanford researchers and others, myofunctional therapy is re-emerging as an integral component of a multidisciplinary approach in the treatment of breathing issues during sleep, as well as a component of orthodontic treatment to encourage optimal craniofacial development and prevent orthodontic relapse.

I think my child has an OMD… what can I do?

The place to start is with your pediatric dentist, pediatrician, ENT physician, sleep physician or pulmonologist. Many medical and dental school programs are beginning to incorporate screening for these issues.

What is the relationship between OMDs and oral habits?

The American Academy of Pediatric Dentistry developed guidelines in 2013 designed to help dentists make decisions during dental visits on practical and timely information about a child's oral habits, including digit and object sucking, bruxism (tooth grinding), tongue thrusting, and nail biting, which should be addressed before correcting crowded or crooked teeth and/or a bad bite, and undesirable facial growth. We advise that patients with these habits be treated or referred for appropriate treatment, whether the patient is age 2 or age 14. Improvement in the dental structure will help with achieving a better bite, proper oral function, and a beautiful face and smile. As a result, a child will grow up with harmonious facial features and properly functioning dentition. Your dentist or pediatric dental specialist has been advised by these guidelines to screen for these oral habits.

Nasal breathing versus mouth breathing… is there a difference?

Yes, and the difference is significant. To mouth breathe, the mouth must be open with the tongue resting low. These dysfunctional oral rest postures of the lips and tongue encourage a multitude of growth and development problems in children, as well as overall health problems. Simply put… if the tongue does not habitually rest on the palate and a child breathes through his mouth, craniofacial development is negatively impacted. Children with dysfunctional oral rest postures and who mouth breathe are more likely to have crowded teeth, small jaws, inadequate tongue room, large tonsils and adenoids, gingivitis, dental caries, and long face syndrome. Additionally, they may also be at greater risk for a wide range of health problems such as allergies, asthma, and disordered breathing issues during sleep, including obstructive sleep apnea. Additionally, nasal breathing confers numerous health benefits that mouth breathing does not.

Breathing through the nose filters the air to remove particulates and allergens, and warms and humidifies the air. The paranasal sinuses produce a gas called nitric oxide, a potent vasodilator that is lethal to both bacteria and viruses when air is inhaled through the nose. Nitric oxide also facilitates increased oxygen absorption by the blood, so mouth breathers actually deliver less oxygen to their own blood than nasal breathers.

What are the signs that may indicate my child might have a breathing problem during sleep?

Snoring, long pauses between breaths, audible breathing through the mouth, grinding and/or clenching of teeth, sweating during sleep, bedwetting, night terrors, consistently restless sleep, difficulty waking, and dry mouth in the morning are symptoms that may indicate your child is experiencing a breathing problem during sleep that warrants further investigation.

Daytime symptoms may also be present. A recent longitudinal study confirmed a strong and persistent association between a child's sleep-disordered breathing symptoms and their behavior. Karen Bonuck, PhD, a professor in the Department of Pediatrics at Albert Einstein College of Medicine, conducted the largest study to date that provides evidence that behavior issues such as inattention, hyperactivity, anxiety, depression, peer problems, and conduct problems may only become apparent years later.[107] Babies demonstrating symptoms between 6 and 18 months of age have 40 to 50% increased behavioral morbidity by age 7. Because of the serious and long-term implications of these findings, we now recommend evaluating for sleep-related breathing symptoms beginning in the first year of life.

How can I tell if my child has an orofacial myofunctional disorder (OMD)?

There are many signs that may indicate a child has an OMD. Strong indicators that an OMD may exist include an open mouth posture; mouth breathing; crowded teeth; a narrow palate; small jaws; a protruding tongue visible at rest, during eating, and/or during speech; dental open bite; dental crossbites; chronic nasal congestion; chronic drooling or difficulty managing one's saliva; kissing tonsils; forward head posture; teeth grinding (both awake and during sleep); and dark circles under the eyes.

My school-age child still sucks her thumb. Is this really a problem? If so, how can I help her stop?

Anything that interferes with the relation between the tongue and the palate is a problem, and thumbs can create big problems! Low muscle tone is associated with thumbsucking, and sucking habits can lead to compensating muscle dysfunction that may interfere with chewing, swallowing, and dental and craniofacial development. Orofacial myofunctional therapists are the experts when it comes to habit elimination for thumbsucking. If your child is still sucking her thumb after age four years, and your attempts to help her stop have been unsuccessful, it is time to seek professional help to minimize further damage. The earlier the better!

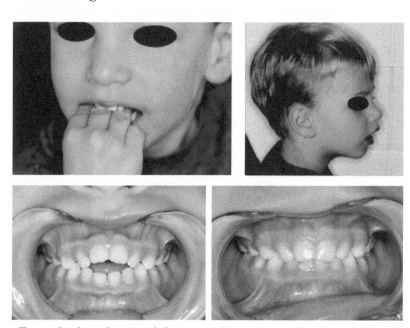

Example of myofunctional therapy with a 2.5 year-old male with a hand biting habit. Results were accomplished in three sessions over three months.

Why is chewing so important?

We have jaws, and we are meant to chew! Unfortunately, today's modern lifestyle has shifted to a diet consisting primarily of highly processed and refined foods, which has reduced our need to chew. Think of the chewing required to eat a whole, raw apple compared with the amount of chewing necessary to consume a dish of applesauce. Whole foods in their natural, unrefined state require more muscle activity to adequately chew and swallow them. More muscle activity means increased optimal growth and development for a child. Anthropologists who study skulls are finding that we have smaller jaws and, consequently, smaller airways than our ancestors of just a few hundred years ago, lending evidence of the epigenetic effects of our modern soft diet and lifestyle.

What does it mean to have a tongue-tie or restricted tongue?

On the underside of the tongue is a soft tissue structure called the lingual frenum that connects the tongue to the floor of the mouth. This is a normal structure, but if the frenum is tight or is attached in a way that restricts movement or mobility of the tongue, the tongue may not be able to access and/or rest on the palate. Often referred to as "tongue-tie," a restricted tongue typically finds a low resting position on the floor of the mouth and can contribute to many orofacial myofunctional disorders (OMDs). A successful outcome with myofunctional therapy requires the ability of the tongue to comfortably access and rest on the palate. If the tongue is restricted, a surgical procedure called a frenectomy can be performed to release a restricted lingual frenum and permit greater mobility and tongue functions. Myofunctional therapy is also essential to the success of a frenectomy procedure and should be incorporated into the postoperative care plan, as it aids in maintaining the full release during the healing process and retrains the tongue to functionally correct rest postures and muscle patterns. The absence of appropriate wound care and myofunctional therapy immediately

217

following surgery often results in a fibrotic reattachment of the released tissues.

Can orofacial myofunctional therapy help adults?

Absolutely. Research continues to validate the benefits of myofunctional therapy for adults. In 2015, Stanford researcher Macario Camacho, MD, and his team published a review of current research in the Sleep Research Society journal *Sleep*, titled "Myofunctional Therapy to Treat OSA."[108] The researchers concluded that myofunctional therapy decreases AHI (Apnea-Hypopnea Index, a measure that indicates the severity of sleep apnea) by approximately 50% in adults and 62% in children, and that snoring and sleepiness outcomes improved in adults following myofunctional therapy. Camacho's review of the research concludes that myofunctional therapy may be a recommended adjunctive therapy in the treatment of obstructive sleep apnea.

How does one obtain credible information and advice on OMDs and OMT therapy programs?

Every person's case is different and unique and can only be properly addressed by a qualified professional during an in-person evaluation. Social media and other Internet sources may not provide accurate or reliable information. More information on myofunctional organizations may be found in the Resources section.

CHAPTER 24

Chiropractic Care

Marty C. Lovvorn, DC

W hy would someone take a baby to a chiropractor? Providers often hear some version of this question. This chapter addresses those questions and others related to chiropractic care. Care for babies, children, and adults will be discussed, as well as how seemingly unrelated issues such as neck pain, neck tension, shoulder pain, and headaches can be related to a tongue-tie.

The number of people seeking chiropractic care for their children and themselves has increased in recent years. It is likely that families seek the advice of their pediatrician or primary care physician with regard to the scope of care and the usefulness of chiropractic care. It is important for parents and other providers to have some helpful information about the benefits of chiropractic care for their patients. Chiropractors in the United States have become the third largest group of healthcare professionals (after physicians and dentists) who have primary contact with patients.[111] According to a 1994 survey, chiropractors were the alternative practitioners most often consulted by pediatric patients.[112] Although most adults (85%) consult chiropractors for musculoskeletal conditions, children frequently visit chiropractors for issues ranging from respiratory concerns to ear/nose/throat issues, and even behavioral concerns. More importantly, a growing number of children and parents alike are seeking chiropractic services for preventative care. In 1993, the American Chiropractic Association reported that 8% of chiropractic patients were younger than 16 years of age, and the National Board of Chiropractic Examiners reported that 10% were younger than 17 years. This equates to approximately 20 million pediatric chiropractic visits annually.[112] The number of children visiting chiropractic offices is substantial and has continued to increase since those figures were published.

When some people hear about chiropractic care for babies, their first image is of a chiropractor taking their fragile newborn and cracking or manipulating the neck in unnatural positions. This image couldn't be further from the truth! Chiropractic care for babies is gentle and painless, and babies often seem more relaxed and restful following treatments. The chiropractor usually begins by taking a history of current symptoms, feeding patterns, and general demeanor, and wants to know about the birth; the first misalignment can begin as the baby is delivered. The baby is then assessed for any subtle abnormalities in cranial shape, muscle tone, and/or joint movements. If a vertebra is found to be out of proper alignment, a gentle pressure is applied to encourage optimal spinal movement. The adjustment is not like that for an adult, where you often hear pops and cracks. The adjustments for babies require steady, gentle pressure applied with only the fingertips. They are similar to checking the ripeness of an avocado or tomato at the grocery store. Following their adjustments, babies are typically able to turn their necks more freely to both sides, allowing nursing issues to improve. Also, babies will often become relaxed, have a break in colic symptoms, or have bowel movements. Why do these things take place? The spinal bones or vertebrae surround and protect the spinal cord, which is composed of billions of nerve fibers that go all throughout the body. These nerves serve as the roads or pathways for the brain to connect with the body. Although most people only think about nerves in the context of pain, that is only a small fraction of the nerve function. The nerves are also responsible for the important things in life—like breathing and bowel movements.

If one vertebra is out of alignment, it can put pressure on the nerve and cause dysfunction. When this happens, the baby is in a state of stress and not relaxation. The most common misalignments in babies and infants occur in the upper parts of their necks or cervical spines, which can send their bodies into "fight-or-flight" sympathetic responses. By relaxing the nervous system, chiropractic adjustments allow babies' bodies to function as intended and prevent unwanted issues such as poor digestion and constipation, poor head control, difficulty nursing (especially if one side is more difficult than another), and general fussiness.

How does a baby's neck get out of alignment?

As is the case with adults, misalignment is rarely caused by major events, but is instead the result of repetitive minor traumas caused by daily activities. Common things like sleeping in car seats or carriers, or even the ways mothers prefer to hold their babies can all cause the vertebrae to misalign. Actually, many of the developmental milestones of the first 2 years can all lead to the need for babies to be checked regularly. These include learning to sit up, beginning to crawl, and pulling up to stand, as well as falling frequently during early walking. For newborns, their positions in the womb, difficult or extended labors, interventions such as vacuum extractions, forceps use, or even Cesarean sections can put forces on their necks and heads that are traumatic to fragile babies.

With the emergence of research on the safety and efficacy of chiropractic care for treating common pediatric symptoms such as breastfeeding issues, colic, reflux, and ear infections, many people are now seeking chiropractic care for these symptoms first. Whereas there is an increase in published research focusing on resolution of breastfeeding issues utilizing chiropractic treatment, there is very little addressing the root cause of these symptoms.[113] One of the items that must be addressed by the chiropractor is the potential for a tongue-tie.

How do you find a chiropractor for infants?

Not all chiropractors see infants or children, so it is important to assess whether the chiropractor you are seeing is comfortable treating babies. Some specialize in athletes, whereas others are more centered on family care. Typically, a chiropractor who sees many pregnant women will likely assess and adjust infants as well. Calling the office beforehand and asking if they routinely treat infants can be helpful. If the receptionist says, "Oh yes, we love seeing babies," that's probably a good sign. If they have to put you on hold to ask someone in the back, it is probably not the best idea to take your infant to that office because they don't see them often. A referral from a lactation consultant can be helpful if you're not sure about chiropractors in your area. Another source of referrals can be moms' groups, either in person or on social media websites such as Facebook. Many in the tongue-tie-specific groups will have sought out a bodyworker such as a chiropractor or craniosacral therapist, and they can give a recommendation for someone who is not only familiar with treating infants but also with tongue-tie issues.

How does a tongue-tie affect breastfeeding, torticollis, and head shape, or cause headaches?

It may seem strange that there could be a connection between a tiny string under the tongue and all of these secondary issues arising in the head, neck, and shoulders. However, the muscles and connective tissue or fascia are intricately connected from the mouth and jaw down to the collarbone and sternum. Even though there are multiple layers of cervical fascia, which can all be involved, the most likely to be adversely affected in tongue-tie is the investing layer of cervical fascia, with connections from the mandible to the hyoid bone, sternocleidomastoid muscles, and trapezius muscles, to name a few. Abnormal stresses on these tissues cause asymmetry, leading to many common presenting symptoms in babies, children and even adults.

Torticollis, also referred to as "wry neck" or cervical dystonia, is a musculoskeletal condition characterized by the inability to turn the head equally from right to left due to tight muscles or fascia on one side. This condition may lead to an array of symptoms in babies and children, including difficulty breastfeeding, tilting of the chin to one side, and a disposition of one shoulder being higher than the other. For adults with torticollis, neck pain, headaches, forward head posture, and tight muscles in the neck and upper shoulders are most common. Therefore, patients commonly present with discomfort in the neck or shoulders from issues arising in the mouth. Unfortunately, not all chiropractors are trained to look for tongue-ties as a potential cause.

A quick word about plagiocephaly. This condition describes a flat or misshapen head. It affects many infants and refers to an asymmetric shape of the cranium (skull bone). It is a condition in which one or more of the sutures (or joints) in an infant's skull prematurely fuse by turning into bone. Even though it can be caused by many factors, it is often due to a combination of the baby's position in the womb, a premature birth, a multiple birth (twins, triplets, etc.), torticollis, use of car seats, and even sleeping on the back. The American Academy of Pediatrics still recommends back sleeping to prevent SIDS; however, tummy time and rotating the head are critical activities used to help babies avoid developing flat spots on the backs of their heads. Chiropractic and craniosacral therapies can be helpful in treating children with plagiocephaly. Some children with moderate or severe cases may need cranial bands or helmets to help reshape the head.

Muscle imbalance issues can affect people at a wide variety of ages. Headaches arising from the neck are caused by neck dysfunction, typically of the upper cervical spine. Although the exact cause of a headache might be unclear and may involve several contributing factors, this particular symptom is commonly associated with muscle imbalance.[114] These muscular imbalances are likely the result of taut and tender fibers in the cervical region involving many of the same muscles affected by long-standing

223

tongue-tie issues. This pattern of muscle imbalance often creates joint dysfunction at the base of the skull and first vertebra (atlas). A tongue-tie could be a contributing factor. A tongue-tie release may help decrease the frequency or severity of headaches and migraines.

Adults are the most common patients seen in a traditional chiropractic office. Adults with pain or tension in their necks and/or shoulders who seem unable to hold their adjustments and need to visit the chiropractor often should consider having evaluations for tongue-ties. If the adult also had speech or feeding difficulties as a child, or currently has trouble with speech, swallowing meat, or taking pills, then a higher index of suspicion for a potential tongue-tie is warranted. Additionally, headaches and poor sleep, such as sleep apnea, lots of movement during sleep, waking easily, or trouble falling asleep, can point to a potential tongue-tie issue.

In both the younger and the older patient, the identification and release of a tongue tie brings almost instant functional improvement. Once the tongue has been released, the chiropractor should assess again and treat if needed, to ensure proper vertebral alignment. Craniosacral therapy should also be considered in conjunction to help reduce fascial adhesions. From the perspective of the chiropractic practitioner, a noticeable increase in range of motion and reduced neck tension can be expected, as the tongue-tie release causes fascial adhesions to release and muscles to relax as well.

If you notice that you or your child are not holding your chiropractic adjustments (you need to go frequently, and seem always to be out of alignment in the same location), or often complain of neck pain, tension in the neck, or poor sleep, then you should have a high degree of suspicion that one of you has a tongue-tie. If these issues are combined with speech difficulties, feeding difficulties, or a history of nursing or bottle-feeding issues in infancy, then an evaluation with a trained tongue-tie provider should be pursued.

CHAPTER 25

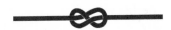

Bodywork, Neurodevelopment, and TummyTime!

Michelle Emanuel, OTR/L, NBCR, CST, CIMI, RYT200

odyworker is an umbrella term used to describe any professional with a hands-on license to touch, who works with the body to effect therapeutic change. Another word for bodywork is manual therapy. Typically, bodywork or soft tissue manual therapy is done through different types and intensities of palpation and touch with the hands, tools or instruments, depending upon the specific professional. A bodyworker, or someone who does manual therapy, is first licensed as an occupational therapist, physical therapist, chiropractor, osteopath (both physician and nonphysician), or licensed massage therapist, among others. In addition to these credentials, most professionals take many hours of advanced training and continuing medical education courses to expand their expertise and treatment techniques.

Bodywork is not simply one modality. There are many types of bodywork to choose from, and your choices are usually dictated by geographical location and the professionals available in your area. Some examples of bodywork modalities/tools are craniosacral therapy (CST), myofascial release (MFR), acupressure, acupuncture, massage, therapeutic skin movement in pediatrics (TSMP), sacral occipital technique (SOT), craniosacral fascial therapy (CFT), and many others. There are mostly similarities among these modalities, and it's preferable to determine what resources and professionals exist in your area, rather than seeking a specific type of treatment modality. One of the most important similarities is that the level and intensity of touch and palpation is always gentle, and the pace is always guided by the baby's individual abilities. While certain techniques, handholds, and positions appear similar between babies, the response and the resultant following of the tissues and the baby are where therapeutic change is made. The most important vetting question you have for a bodyworker is: "Are you familiar with and trained to work with babies?" Generally speaking, any manual therapy modality in the hands of a person with baby experience will be helpful, as they all have efficacy and importance. Additionally, they all have an effect on a baby's nervous system, and this is helpful to the whole body.

Other similarities among soft tissue techniques include working with fascia and the skin organ, and engaging the brain and nervous system. Fascia, or connective tissue, is pervasive in the body, connecting muscles to bones and bones to bones, and wrapping muscle bundles and even individual cells. Fascia is a continuous body part from the top of our heads to the tips of our toes. It is composed of collagen, elastin, and ground substance (a watery type of fluid). A tongue-tie is composed of fascia, and this fascia is connected to all the other parts of the body. This is one reason why the tongue has such a powerful effect on how a baby's body is positioned and moves. When releasing a tongue-tie, the release provider is releasing fascia, not muscle. Muscles move the body, and fascia connects the body; it is the interconnected dance between them that dictates how the bones grow, movement happens, and feeding and nursing succeed. When a baby has a tongue-tie release, the fascia/connective tissue is released, which enables the nervous system to direct muscles to move the tongue in wider ranges of motion and with a more optimal and mature sucking pattern.

Why do babies need bodywork?

Aren't babies perfect? I'm often asked these two questions in my private practice and in the Facebook parent support group I administrate. Babies with oral dysfunction and tethered oral tissues have altered tongue function. For a baby, the mouth is the primary sensory and perceptual organ, and its function, or lack thereof, will be reflected in other body parts. A typically developing baby's "best" movement and functional skills come from the mouth, specifically the tongue. Therefore, the baby relies on compensation and adaptive movement rather than optimal movements to sustain nursing and oral function. One example of the structural consequences of a restricted tongue is a high-arch palate.[64] Having a high-arch palate is a less-than-optimal configuration/shape for nasal breathing and sinus development; it promotes hypersensitivity in the oral cavity, and contributes to poor nursing skills, typically by loss of suction or negative pressure generation. Bodywork techniques help the soft tissues of the body slide and glide in tense, restricted, or "sticky" spots. These spots hinder movement and sensorimotor processing, and they benefit from the shifts and changes brought about by gentle manual therapy and bodywork techniques.

Bodyworkers and therapists assist with identification of tethered oral tissues, through the use of validated tools such as the Martinelli protocol[36] and the HATLFF[34] (both previously mentioned) paired with clinical assessment, symptoms, and individual circumstances. Additionally, many professionals have wound care in their scope of practice. This can be helpful for those with active wound management after tongue-tie release. Regardless of the tool used for frenum release (CO_2 laser, diode laser, scissors, scalpel, etc.), the wound needs to heal by secondary intention. This means that rather than sealing up the wound the way it was before release, we want the wound to fill in with new tissue and stay in a diamond-like shape so the newly formed frenum is more flexible. Bodywork techniques that achieve sliding and gliding in the tissues, engaging active movements of the tongue and intentional TummyTime!, assist with an optimal healing process.

Another way bodywork and soft tissue manual therapy can be helpful is with comfort management, both pre- and post-TOTs release. In addition to practicing skin-to-skin contact and minimizing environmental "busy-ness" for you at home, there are several avenues that can be utilized to ease discomfort. These include regulatory activities for baby's nervous system, using touch, gentle hand positions, unwinding movements, rhythm, and movement. These and more help with natural pain relief through feel-good hormones.

To the parents of babies and children undergoing tongue release habilitation process: it's helpful for you to receive some bodywork. While it is a lot easier and less stressful to go through this process with full-team support, it is still stressful. It is not easy for you to learn all this new terminology, make decisions based on new information, do the exercises, learn how to care for the wound and realize that you can't go through it for your baby, but you can be strong, calm and confident. Consider asking who in your area specializes with adults and experience a healing session yourself. Some bodyworkers specialize in babies, children, and adults, so you may not have far to look.

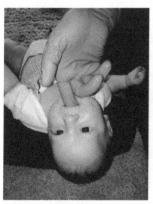 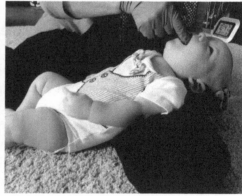

When you take your baby to a bodyworker, expect to find a warm, welcoming environment and a competent and compassionate professional. Most professionals use bodywork on massage tables, balls, tilted surfaces, and the floor to work. A head-to-toe assessment will be performed in tune with your baby's natural rhythms. In addition to noting physical considerations, such as tense areas, areas with armoring and protective responses, and decreased tissue movement, the practitioner will assess and treat nervous system dysregulation to maximize the baby's responses to treatment. This may include relaxing the baby's nervous system and tissues or encouraging more energy and vitality, depending upon the unique needs of your baby. Gentle passive movements and, often, oral, primitive, and postural reflexes as well as other movements are utilized to promote natural alignment and balance in the baby's body. Bodyworkers tend to use slow, gentle movements to nudge tissues into natural alignment and soft tissue integrity. This has a positive effect on the whole body as well. Sometimes areas of the body feel like a kinked garden hose, and they need to be moved to open up and let the water pass through.

Most babies benefit from 2 to 6 sessions; however, more may be necessary depending upon factors such as follow-through with home programming, a baby's level of compromise at initiation of treatment, and the speed of progress and changes noted. Initially, the baby may be seen 1 to 2 times per week, gradually tapering off with greater time between sessions.

What should I expect after a bodywork session?

There are a wide range of responses to bodywork, including sleeping, pooping a bit more than usual, increased movement, improved latch and nursing skills, and sometimes even obvious physical or structural changes, such as a flat spot not looking as flat, or an asymmetrical or uneven facial expression becoming more symmetrical. Other times, baby may cry briefly or be more active, and this can cause some nervous system dysregulation. Most of the time, there is a favorable response to bodywork. If you do not feel comfortable or something feels not quite right, please speak to the bodyworker or perhaps find another practitioner who may be a better fit. After all, it's not just about the tools or modalities being used, but also the bodyworker's therapeutic presence and ability to interact with the baby and your family, which also make huge contributions to the outcome.

Neurodevelopment and Therapeutic Intentional TummyTime!

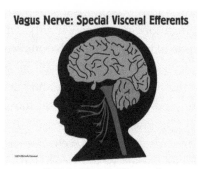

©2016 Michelle Emanuel

Cranial nerves are a set of 12 nerves located in the primitive brainstem. These nerves provide sensory and motor capabilities to the muscles of facial expression, the tongue, larynx (voice box), pharynx (throat), soft palate, head and shoulder muscles, inner ear, the jaw and associated temporomandibular joints, and muscles and sensory nerves that equip the eyes. All of these body parts are of paramount importance for a baby fresh out of the womb. Cranial nerve dysfunction (CND) is a term used to describe a baby's functional deficits, with a specific emphasis on cranial nerves. It isn't a diagnosis; it's a way for trained professionals to view a baby's functional status, guide the timing of release, and determine the level of therapeutic needs. Babies with TOTs can be categorized as having mild, moderate, or significant cranial nerve dysfunction. The level of severity is determined by symptoms, such as asymmetries, gastrointestinal symptoms (reflux, gas, aerophagia, etc.), airway compromise (squeaky breathing, etc.), vocal prosody (quality and resonance of baby's voice), facial expressivity, and much more.

A key developmental component necessary for all babies is postural control and development. A baby must practice negotiating gravity, active and passive movements, and reflexive and spontaneous movements, all the while needing to nurse effectively enough to gain weight, grow, feel connected, and safe. For babies, one of the important positions for postural and neurodevelopment is prone play or "tummy time," a term which should be familiar. Tummy time is time a baby spends on his or her tummy on a firm flat surface, usually the floor. All pediatricians recognize and value tummy time as integral to a baby's development.

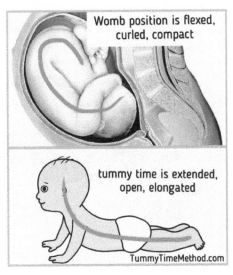

Womb position is flexed, curled, compact

tummy time is extended, open, elongated

TummyTimeMethod.com

Babies transform from the helpless newborn period, to crawling, to pulling to stand, and typically begin walking within one year of extrauterine life. The breast crawl, baby's innate ability to crawl up mother's body and latch independently within 1 to 3 hours after being born is a testament to how prone play or tummy time equips babies for surviving and thriving. The breast crawl is not possible when babies are placed on their backs, or the supine position, and babies will not survive or thrive in this position after birth. Babies, especially in the precrawling period to age 3, have a rapidly developing nervous system. An older child or adult, however, has leveled off and reached a relatively stable phase, although neuroplasticity and change are possible throughout the entire lifespan. At birth, human babies require the most support and assistance with positioning and movements when compared with all other mammals. Babies rely on parents and caregivers to put them in every position they are in. For example, if a baby is placed in a swing for sleep with the head to the preferred side and more pressure on a flat spot, the baby cannot adjust herself to derail further damage. The term "fourth trimester" has been given to the first 12 weeks of extrauterine life to highlight the continued neurodevelopmental maturation and processes required by human infants beyond a typical 40-week gestation.

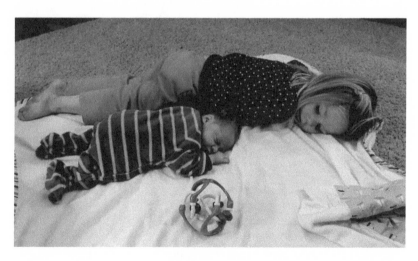

Babies rely on their parents and caregivers to put them in positions and introduce them to varied movements to challenge and stimulate the nervous system for optimal neurodevelopmental progression. Babies develop in a cephalocaudal manner, meaning they develop in a head (cephalo) to tail (caudal) order: head first, tail last. Whereas babies without compromised oral function and restrictions who are held a lot and worn (both are forms of tummy time) receive enough stimulation and input from these activities, babies with tethered oral tissues need specific, therapeutic, intentional tummy time experiences to properly address and remediate oral functional deficits.

In 1992, the American Academy of Pediatrics (AAP) rolled out two important recommendations for babies. Called "Back to Sleep" and "Tummy to Play," these initiatives highlighted the need for intentional tummy time in a back-sleeping culture. In 2011, the AAP reiterated the need for tummy time, specifically stating that it is needed to prevent plagiocephaly, or flattening of baby's head. The current incidence of plagiocephaly is 46.6%, so roughly *half* of all babies are affected.[115] Another clinical finding that has remained consistent in my practice over the past 10 years is the link between TOTs and head flattening (i.e., plagiocephaly, brachycephaly, scaphocephaly, and other random head-molding patterns). Again, this has not been formally studied or published. It is a result of seeing the same restrictions, issues, and patterns over years of experience, combined with what I know about optimal infant oral development.

Tummy time is integral to baby's neurodevelopment and oral feeding skills, because when a baby is in this position, the whole body is engaged in weight shifts and movement, which support tongue and oral function. In utero, babies spend their time curled up or flexed forward, with limited movements into straightening the body, also called extension. From birth to about 9 months, babies spend their time straightening or extending their body, and this is best done in the tummy-time position. Tummy time helps baby learn to move and control movements in the gravity field. Baby's first big developmental goal and achievement, aside from bonding/attachment and nursing, is head control. One tummy-time study revealed significant differences in head control between babies who engaged in tummy time and those who did not.[116] For a baby to develop head control, the tongue needs to have optimal function; this includes range of motion, strength, and endurance. Tongue-tie limits all three of these parameters and hinders oral function, and many times it hinders nursing, although some tongue-tied babies do nurse adequately without pain or discomfort.

So let's just get all the babies in tummy time, right? Yes! However, there are a few snags and difficulties for babies with tethered oral tissues. Your own baby may have a dislike for tummy time or you may have heard that other babies "hate" tummy time. I am here to assure you that babies do not hate anything, but they will signal distress or discomfort when applicable. The interesting thing to note is that babies with TOTs have particular difficulties with tummy-time experiences, which range from physical to functional restrictions.

Here's an exercise that can help make this point clearer: Pull your tongue down into the floor of your mouth as if you have a tongue tie, then lie down on your tummy and try to lift and turn your head; try to push up with your arms and lengthen the front of your neck and shoulders. This is a small part of the unique tummy-time challenges TOTs babies face. And I haven't even mentioned nervous system dysregulation, head-turning preference and torticollis, head flattening (plagiocephaly, brachycephaly, scaphocephaly), gastrointestinal issues (such as reflux, gas, and aerophagia), and airway compromise.

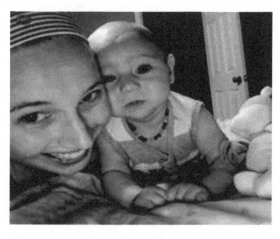

After working with many babies who struggled secondary to physical and functional limitations and restrictions, I developed the TummyTime!™ Method (TTM), which is a simple yet powerfully effective way to help babies and parents connect and LOVE tummy time. In addition to this, TTM was developed specifically:

» To promote nervous system regulation—how baby calms, settles, and soothes
» To decrease reflux
» To promote effective burping and gas release
» To decrease head turning preference or torticollis
» To optimize tongue and jaw function by eliminating compensations and promoting new, functional movements
» To elicit, utilize, and integrate oral, primitive, and postural reflexes
» To promote whole-body active and passive movements

TTM takes it further than just getting baby in the tummy-time or prone position; it's a treatment approach utilizing the prone position with specific intent to calm the nervous system and optimize cranial nerve function, which leads to optimal oral and neurodevelopmental progress and abilities. TTM also problem solves to help babies who struggle in other developmental areas, such as head control, turning head to both sides, engaging in relaxed body postures a majority of the time, etc.

While many people understand the connection between tummy time and tongue-tie based on these types of discussions, there aren't any specific published studies at this time. However, a recent study reveals that babies who cannot push themselves up with extended (straight) arms in tummy time at 6 months of age have developmental lags or delays when compared with babies who can push up on extended arms.[117]

To be effective at pushing up with arms, a baby needs experience with tummy time. Often very little time has been spent in tummy time, and most tongue-tied babies either push up too vigorously and get upset, or they avoid pushing up with their arms.

This directly impacts development, including oral functional skills. Additionally, many babies with tethered oral tissues are either extended or arched backward, which also results in head lag when pulled to sit or flexed with a head-forward posture. Both of these patterns, extended and flexed, reflect an imbalance or dysregulation of postural integrity.

In my professional experience, TTM is effective at reducing compensation patterns from a tongue-tie. I also reliably see increased strength, endurance, and function of oral and postural skills. Having a reliable home-based therapy that you do with your baby on a daily basis contributes to therapeutic changes and progress. Doing TTM with your baby in between lactation and bodywork sessions supports and maintains exercises, activities and direct hands-on support provided during therapy sessions. Your baby is at home with you 7 days a week, 24 hours a day, whereas your baby is with a lactation consultant or bodyworker for 1 to 2 hours a couple of times a week. It is worthwhile to have TTM in your repertoire; find a local professional to help or check out my YouTube channel (search Michelle Emanuel).

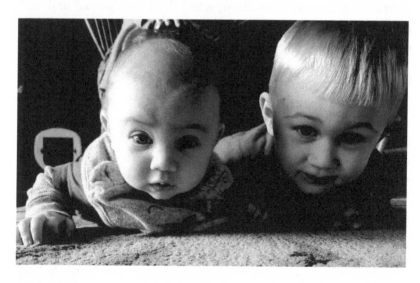

In 2015, I completed an informal study in my office, in which I assessed 20 babies using a validated OT/PT postural responses in gravity assessment. An experienced and qualified dentist diagnosed all 20 babies with posterior tongue-tie, and all of them had undergone a tongue-tie release before my assessment. I had expected to find some postural delays because of my experiences; however, I was surprised to find that 17 of 20 babies scored 2 standard deviations below the norm. This means that an overwhelming majority of babies with posterior tie had delayed postural responses to caregiving activities. This was concerning to me as a neurodevelopmental expert because I more fully understood the challenges babies with ties were facing. I also was concerned because not one of the babies had been referred to me by their pediatricians. Because this study was not done within the rigors of a scientific or medical institution, I cannot make broad claims about this, but I can say that we need to take a closer look at a possible link between tongue-tie, posture, and developmental skills. A strong developmental link exists between tongue function and postural development and integrity. Yet here is the good news: 15 of 17 scored within a normal range within 6 weeks by using the 4 Part Functional Movement Protocol (FMP), which includes:

1. Reducing or avoiding the use of containers (infant seats, swings, and other baby equipment) and containment (swaddling and other restrictive items)
2. Implementation of TummyTime!™ Method and promoting optimal movements through various developmental activities
3. Promoting changes in activities of daily living that contribute to normalization of oral function
4. Ensuring optimal position during nighttime sleep and daytime napping, which contributes to optimal oral function

How much therapeutic, intentional tummy time do babies with TOTs need?

Rather than focus on the quantity of tummy time, focus on the *quality* of tummy and floor time experiences. As babies have repeated pleasurable and connected experiences, comfort and ease help baby enjoy and even seek tummy-time experiences. Tummy time doesn't last a long time—just 5 minutes a few times a day is helpful to begin. Based on my experience, babies are more successful and engaged in tummy time when introduced frequently for short periods of time. Get down on the floor with your baby, sing familiar songs, talk, and connect with your baby. These repeated experiences with you help your baby adapt and mature developmentally.

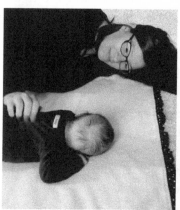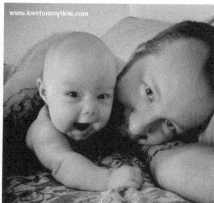

TTM TIP: If you are struggling to do frequent, short tummy-time sessions, simply roll baby into tummy time for a minute following each diaper change. Over the course of the day, this will add up, and every little bit helps.

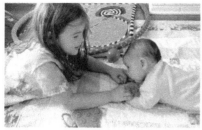 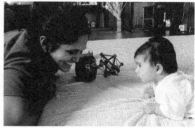

When does tummy time start?

Babies benefit from starting tummy time right from birth. The first 2 weeks of life is spent primarily on the chest of a parent or caregiver; however, after that, a blanket on the floor is the best place to engage with baby for tummy time. So, what do you do if you haven't started tummy time yet and your baby is much older? Just start where you are today. Do several short sessions of fun tummy-time play.

It is essential for therapeutic professionals to collaborate and communicate with lactation consultants and release providers. This does not necessarily mean they work for the same business or agency, but they work in a team approach, communicate, and make appropriate referrals to provide comprehensive care for your baby and family.

What are some alternative tummy-time positions?

- » Boppy pillow
- » Over your lap
- » Over your arm
- » On a physioball or beach ball
- » Babywearing (front and back carries)

Is tummy time safe?

Yes! You are always with your baby during tummy-time activities. Tummy time is the beginning of how you and baby play together. Interacting and playing together while on the floor for tummy time is fun, safe, and a great way to spend time together.

Other populations:

Tummy time or prone play isn't just for babies. Toddlers, preschoolers, school-age children, adolescents, and adults of all ages benefit from time on their tummy. Some people go to exercise classes and some do yoga or Pilates; others attend developmental movement and dance classes, which emphasize belly-to-earth movements. Regardless, we all need to experience weight bearing, weight shifting, and rotational movements in our bodies for optimal health and wellness.

CHAPTER 26

———— ∞ ————

Adults

Often adults don't realize they are tongue-tied until some event involving their baby or child causes them to think about their own mouth. These adults have usually seen many healthcare providers, but no one has checked underneath the tongue. Sometimes an adult patient presents for an examination and says they had their tongue clipped as a baby. If this is the case, they are asked to lift their tongue to their palate, with their mouth wide open, to see how highly the tongue can elevate. Many times the tongue can barely elevate one inch, when in fact it should almost reach or be touching the palate. This is a quick screening test. Further evaluation and questions can then take place to determine if the adult patient is having symptoms warranting a release.

A search on PubMed for "tongue-tie and adults," "tongue-tie and TMJ issues," and "tongue tie and migraines" returns few results. Only one article discusses treating tongue-tie in adults. In 1993, Mukai discussed treatment of 38 adult patients with congenital ankyloglossia, with most of them having a Class III jaw relationship (underbite) irregular tooth alignment, or a high-arched palate. [118] They also reported subjective symptoms of "stiffness of the shoulders, a cold feeling in the extremities, an obstructed feeling in the throat, insomnia, fatigue, dry skin, irritability and/or anxiety, and nervousness."[118] The subjects reported that all of these symptoms improved postoperatively. In addition, the objective symptoms that improved included "snoring, muscle cramps, difficulty in playing wind instruments, [and] hoarseness."[118] Incorrect articulation did not improve postoperatively, likely because speech therapy is required to retrain the muscles and compensations after decades of incorrect and restricted muscle activity and habits. While tongue-ties have been thoroughly studied in the infant population, they have not been studied in the adult population, but hopefully this will change.

Healthcare providers are rarely educated about the issues that can accompany tongue-ties in adults, such as neck tension or pain, shoulder tension or pain, TMJ pain, migraine and other headaches, and sleep disorders. Reflux and digestive issues can continue into adulthood if food is not properly processed due to ineffective chewing. Sometimes reflux results from aerophagia (swallowing air with food or liquid). Air that enters the GI tract must eventually go back out, either through the mouth or through the rectum. Many people are able to stop their reflux medications shortly after having their tongue-ties released. Nighttime grinding and clenching of teeth (bruxism) are also often alleviated after a tongue-tie release and subsequent myofunctional therapy. A patient's posture may improve. Before the procedure, the patient may hold his head in a forward position, whereas afterward, he may be able to hold his head more normally, in a neutral position.

A 37 year-old woman recently presented with a history of terrible stuttering since age 4. She had been to therapist after therapist, trying to find someone who could help with her debilitating speech impediment. In addition to struggling with her speech, she also had neck and shoulder pain. She never thought about whether she might have a tongue-tie, but after her baby had its tongue-tie treated, she was examined with that in mind. Her tongue elevated about halfway when she opened her mouth as widely as she could. She had a posterior tongue-tie that was not easily visible, so it had never been identified. After her tongue function and her speech were assessed, the patient was offered a tongue-tie release. The procedure took about 1 minute, with no sutures, bleeding, or sedation. After the procedure, she was able to say the Pledge of Allegiance with minimal effort and significantly less stuttering. A week later, she came back for a follow-up visit and reported that she still struggled with her speech, but she was having more good days than bad ones, her neck pain was much better, and she now had hopes of eventually speaking normally. Her husband and mother noticed an immediate difference in her speech.

This story is not an isolated event. It is the story of many patients in many different offices across the country. Each patient has a unique story. One mother (of a baby who was tied) who came for a release had been the youngest patient ever treated at a large research university hospital migraine clinic at the age of 5. She had suffered from migraines and neck pain her whole life. Her tongue-tie was easily visualized and extended almost to the tip of her tongue. After the release, she immediately felt the tension leave her neck and shoulders. She was finally able to turn her head without pain while driving. Her migraines decreased in severity and frequency. Dramatic improvements in basic activities of daily living are common. If the right questions are asked, a provider may discover the related symptoms and tie the pieces together (pun intended). But often, providers address other problems and do not ever notice the tongue-tie. For example, if a person has TMJ (jaw joint) problems, he might talk to his dentist and get a mouth guard because he is suspected of grinding his teeth at night. However, the joint problems may be due to a tongue-tie (or another factor) causing sleep problems and he is grinding because he is sleeping poorly and not getting enough oxygen to his brain. The brain in turn tries to wake him up by causing him to grind his teeth and open the airway. This is not the cause of all tooth grinding or bruxism, but sleep should be evaluated in kids and adults who are grinding their teeth at night. A person may use a night guard, which may help, or he might be prescribed a muscle relaxant to calm the muscles and limit the grinding, but the cause has only been masked. If these are unsuccessful, any manner of treatments for TMJ may be initiated, and the patient may still have issues. Typically, even with all of these treatments from various practitioners, no one has fully evaluated the tongue, which could be tied down. People who suffer from TMJ pain may have improvement in their symptoms if they have tongue ties and these are addressed.

I myself had my tongue tie treated in adulthood. I had nursing difficulties as a baby and speech issues as a child. These continued through adolescence and into adulthood. I needed a maxillary or palatal expander and had braces three times. I had jaw surgery to correct an underbite from an underdeveloped upper jaw, and had joint surgery in my TMJ to prevent joint issues in the future, which, I was told, could arise after jaw surgery. I had a night guard to keep me from destroying my teeth when I was grinding and clenching them every night. Then I was prescribed a muscle relaxant to help stop the grinding. After the jaw surgery, I had constant sinus infections requiring countless rounds of antibiotics and two sinus surgeries. Malformed sinuses from a non-expanded nasal airway (the palate is the floor of the nasal cavity) can result from a low tongue posture. It was not until I was in dental school that my tongue-tie was discovered by a periodontist because it was causing gum recession, a common finding with tongue-ties. He used a laser, but only released a tiny portion of it, which was right next to the tooth, instead of releasing the large string that was still there after all those years that no one saw (or was trained to identify and treat).

Years later, a lactation consultant brought tongue-ties to my attention after our girls were born and struggled with nursing. After learning everything I could about tongue-ties, including taking courses and performing releases, I had my associate release my tongue with our CO_2 laser. My tongue immediately felt more mobile, making it easier for me to talk and swallow. I could talk faster and speak more clearly, and I no longer tired when talking or reading aloud. My TMJ pain, locking, and popping, which happened daily before the release, went away. Neck tension that I wasn't even aware of also disappeared. I wish it had been discovered and corrected when I was a baby, or even a young child. I saw at least 4 different dentists, 2 speech therapists,

3 different orthodontists, 2 oral surgeons, and 2 pediatricians, and no one identified or treated it.

There are many people who relate similar stories. If this is your story, don't look backward, just move forward. I'm in no way blaming those who saw my mouth, but didn't notice or say anything about the tongue-tie. The problem was a systemic lack of education about the potentially serious effects of tongue-ties across medical and dental specialties. This book is an attempt to encourage others in the academic world to join those of us who treat these patients as we investigate these issues further.

Section 5: What Now?

A fter reading this far, you may have determined that someone you know likely has a tongue-tie. If you're a provider, you might have several patients in mind who could benefit from releases. This section will discuss the steps to choosing release providers and give parents and practitioners some helpful questions to ask potential providers to ensure they are knowledgeable about the latest concepts, and successful performing the procedures with whatever method they currently offer. Later sections on conclusions and best practices will review the highlights and main takeaways for patient treatment and parent knowledge. Ten additional case presentations from newborns to adults will be shared. These illustrate the different symptoms of tongue and lip restrictions and the improvements these patients saw. As always, functions and complaints are more critical than appearances. Finally, the section will conclude with next steps for professionals, a list of resources for parents and providers, and the list of references used in the writing of this book. The Appendix includes templates for practice documents that may be useful to providers in taking histories and doing aftercare. Parents may find the questions on the forms helpful as well since they precisely pinpoint the kinds of functional issues that may be encountered.

CHAPTER 27

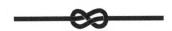

Choosing a Provider

There are many different ways to find a provider who is knowledgeable about tethered oral tissues. If you have a baby with a tongue-tie, it is best to discuss this with your lactation consultant if you have one, and they can point you in the right direction. However, even among lactation consultants, knowledge of and experience with tongue-ties is inconsistent. If you suspect a tongue-tie, let your lactation consultant know. If she thinks it is there, but not a big deal (and you think it may be), reach out to friends or breastfeeding groups. With the rise of social media sites like Facebook, more information than ever is available online. There are groups for tongue-tied babies, tongue-tied kids, and even tongue-tied adults. These groups can be a great resource, but can also cause parents to worry needlessly. Be sure to take these sites with a grain of salt. Look for overall trends and reviews of different providers. The state-specific tongue-tie groups, (like our "Alabama Tongue and Lip Tie Support Group," which has about 1,100 members at the time of this writing), are a great resource for moms with questions about providers (release providers, lactation consultants, bodyworkers, and others). Most states have state-specific tongue-tie groups that are probably the most helpful resources for parents to go to for state-specific information, such as which providers are recommended and available in their area. The largest group (currently around 65,000 members and counting), called Tongue-Tied Babies Support Group, is helpful, but keep in mind these support groups are facilitated by parents and volunteers and do not constitute medical advice. If someone has a bad release experience (which is rare but does happen), other moms might be scared and not seek treatment for their children. It is important to seek out an in-person observation by a TOTs-knowledgeable professional as early as possible, even if travel to another area is required. Remember, you cannot diagnose a lip- or tongue-tie from a photograph alone.

Readers who are not in the United States also have a wide range of available resources, depending on where they are located, such as the Facebook group Infant Tongue-Tie, UK, Ireland, and Europe, which has 4,000 members. Clearly, tongue-ties are not isolated to one particular country or geographic area, and awareness is growing in many parts of the world. The Internet has brought people together as never before and is, for the most part, a helpful community where moms can band together, support each other and give helpful advice. One of the goals of this book is to motivate healthcare providers to disseminate up-to-date information and to include assessments for tongue-ties in their repertoire of newborn and infant exams.

In the Internet age, before people buy things, they check for reviews. Whether they are buying TVs, cars, even meals at restaurants, people want to check Amazon, Facebook, Google, or Yelp to hear what other people have to say. With tongue-tie releases, it is not a bad idea to find out what other people think. However, look for general trends, and don't just focus on one or two reviews. Typically, if providers do many releases, they will have a number of Google reviews, Facebook reviews, or people inside the social media tongue-tie groups who have experienced their care.

It can be hit or miss to ask a hospital or pediatrician for a referral. Pediatricians may refer children to ENTs because they are used to sending their patients to them for tonsils, adenoids, and ear tubes. It may not even cross their mind that a dentist or pediatric dentist can do this procedure. By all means, ask your pediatrician for a referral, but ask questions about where they are sending you, check for reviews online, and ask lactation consultants and other breastfeeding moms in your area. Different providers have different levels of interest in and skill at performing this procedure. For adults, the best place to check is on the Facebook groups or on the so-called preferred provider list for adult providers.

The Preferred Provider List

This resource may be helpful, but it is incomplete and leaves out qualified people who can do the procedure. Overall, it is a step in the right direction, and it is nice that someone took the time to compile all of the information to help parents find a starting point to use when trying to assist their baby or older child. This list is often referred to in Facebook groups as a "preferred provider list," but it shouldn't be confused with a preferred provider organization, or PPO, like an insurance company list. This list is compiled after a provider submits a detailed explanation of her stance on breastfeeding, how she does a release, what a posterior tongue-tie is, what stretching exercises are typically recommended, and other factors that could help determine whether the person asking to be included on the list is up to date with the latest tongue-tie information. It can be found at http://www.tt-lt-support-network.com/, and it has a list of providers for most states and even some other countries. Some states (such as California) have about 25 providers, whereas the state of Alabama has only one. However, there are other good providers in this state, so clearly the list is not complete. It is a good starting point, but it is not the only resource.

Questions to Ask a Provider for Infant Tongue-Tie Release

Once you are at the release provider's office, here are some helpful questions to ask. The first question should be about his experience in treating tongue-ties in people with your condition, whether it is nursing, speech, feeding, etc. Ask about any recent continuing education classes he has taken, whether online or in person, related to tongue-ties. The research and newest thinking regarding this condition are evolving rapidly right now, so he should have attended a course or at the very least viewed an online course within the last few years. Tongue-tie education not adequate in most training programs, so seeking out additional postgraduate information is critical. If you are a provider and are reading this part, it's easy to find courses. Check the Resources section in the back of the book for a list of available courses.

The next question to ask is regarding posterior tongue-tie. Does she treat posterior tongue-ties? Does she know what they are? If you ask her about exercises and she says that aftercare stretching or exercises are unnecessary, or she indicates that they have not developed a protocol for wound management after the procedure, ask follow-up questions or look elsewhere. The wound can quickly grow back together, and that can cause symptoms to come back and potentially require repeat surgery. The provider should be able to tell you what method he uses to release the frenum. If it is a laser, he should know the type and all of the laser safety protocols that need to be followed. For example, he needs to make sure the baby, assistant, doctor, and any observers have laser-specific protective eyewear, the door is closed, and a "Laser in Use" sign must be on the door. There's much more to laser safety, but that's just an example of a few items that should be known and practiced by doctors using a laser.

Another great question to ask providers is whom they recommend for follow-up. Who is on their team? A lactation consultant? Myofunctional therapist? Speech therapist? Bodyworker? Treating tethered oral tissues fully requires a team approach.

If you have an appointment with a dental or medical provider and you have dental or medical insurance, make sure your baby is on the insurance plan by contacting your HR manager or the company directly. Typically, a parent has 30 days to add a new baby to her health or dental insurance policy. After that, she will have to wait until the next open enrollment period to get the baby covered.

The younger the baby is when the release is performed, the better the baby will typically recover. Sometimes a dental plan will cover only one frenectomy at a time (either upper or lower), and often it won't cover the procedure at all because they say it is medical or that it is unnecessary. If your child has symptoms and functional issues from a tongue-tie, don't let a lack of insurance coverage deter you from getting your child needed care. Often beneficial procedures are denied by medical or dental insurance companies for various reasons. Sometimes insurance company denials can be overcome with good documentation of medical necessity. Parents are occasionally forced to choose to do only one procedure when a baby needs two, or they do both and pay an additional amount out of pocket. Typically, it is best to do everything needed at one visit so the baby or child is not subjected to multiple surgical visits. However, if finances or insurance coverage are causing issues, then typically the tongue should be performed first, and then, at the one-week follow-up, the tongue can be checked and the lip can be performed if needed. This sequence is recommended because typically the tongue is the most at fault, and also because it takes the tongue about a week longer to heal than the lip. This will prevent the baby from having to undergo more weeks of aftercare stretches than would otherwise be necessary.

Depending on the state and on insurance company factors, a dentist can sometimes send the claim to the medical insurer, or sometimes she can give the parents a letter so they can submit the claim to the medical insurance company. Most dentists will be able to provide you with dental and medical codes to use when you submit the claim on your own to your dental or medical insurance company, although every insurance plan is different and covers the procedure differently. If you have insurance or financial questions, it is best to call your provider's office to determine in advance what's covered, approximately how much the procedure will cost, and what will be due at the time of the consult. If you're concerned about a tongue-tie, the consultation does not mean you have to do the procedure the same day, and it is best to at least hear what the provider has to say after the baby has been evaluated. Most providers will do the procedure on the same day as the consult, but it is certainly not required.

Providers for Children or Adults with Tongue-Tie

Most of these recommendations for providers and questions to ask providers relate to babies and mothers with nursing issues. It can be harder to find providers who release toddlers' tethered tissues because they are generally uncooperative in the dental chair. It is a quick procedure, about 20 seconds, but they have to be still for those 20 seconds. If it is possible to wait, sometimes it is better to postpone the procedure until the child is more cooperative, which is usually around age four, rather than put the child through sedation or general anesthesia and the stretching exercises. The child might have a difficult time understanding the reason for the stretches or the procedure, but if the procedure can be done when the child is a little older, it might make it easier on the whole family. If a child is gagging when eating, is speech delayed, has poor sleep quality, or having other significant issues at the toddler stage, and there is a tongue-tie, then the benefits may outweigh the risks. Determining whether the child needs the procedure at every age is made on a case-by-case basis. In a toddler, a tongue release should be done either without any sedation or with minimal oral sedation, like midazolam (Versed, similar to Valium). It should only be performed by a provider trained in safe pediatric sedation and experienced in releasing tongue-ties in this age group. Most of the toddlers and preschool children we release are being treated for significant speech and feeding issues, and are rarely sedated. A strong numbing jelly is applied, and they normally cry for the duration of the procedure (around 10 seconds), but then sit up and calm down quickly with minimal distress after getting a balloon and a prize. The stress on the child is similar to that seen after a routine immunization. Often, the parents report that later in the day the child acts as if nothing happened. The child will experience mild-to-moderate discomfort after the procedure for a few days, but their pain is usually controlled with ibuprofen or acetaminophen and a few scoops of ice cream.

Many general dentists, oral surgeons, pediatric dentists, and ENTs release school-age through high school-age children. Young adults and older adults may find it difficult to locate a provider because most pediatricians or pediatric dentists will only treat kids. Often an oral surgeon, general dentist, or ENT is a good choice for an adult release, but be sure to consult the resources above, such as the preferred provider list and the questions to ask, to find someone who is up to date on the latest techniques and research. Using a laser is the preferred route for older children and adults, too. It provides excellent visibility during surgery to ensure a full release, is typically less painful, and it heals quickly.

For older children, I will sometimes place sutures, depending on whether the patient is likely to follow through with postoperative exercises and stretching the wound. If you don't think you can stretch the wound yourself to prevent it healing back together, then sutures (stitches) may be a good option. Keep in mind that sutures limit mobility and function more than a release that is left open and aided with postoperative exercises and myofunctional therapy. Also, just because a dentist or other professional owns a laser, does not mean that they know how to release a tongue properly. Ask questions similar to the infant questions, such as "How often do you do tongue-tie releases?" and "What is your aftercare stretching protocol?" Find out what exercises or myofunctional therapy they recommend, and who is on their team. Again, as with infants, there are a few Facebook pages dedicated to kids and adults with tongue-ties, aptly named Tongue-Tied Kids and Tongue-Tied Adults Support Group, which include lists of providers for adults and kids.

CHAPTER 28

Conclusions and Best Practices

It is a bold statement to say, "This is the way it should be done," and any other way is wrong. So just to be clear, that's not what this section is about. This section lays out our ideas of best practices and our opinion of what seems to work best for babies, adults, and everyone in between. Other methods can be effective and may be preferred by those accustomed to using them. Another way to look at this section is that we have a few key takeaways that we would like to summarize for our readers.

Babies are a vulnerable group of tiny humans that need our help. Thankfully, there is literature published that supports helping these babies, although more research and more widespread knowledge of the current research are needed. Babies need a team approach to management. Beginning on day one of life, the OB/GYN, pediatrician, nursing staff, and lactation consultant should work together to perform a preliminary assessment of the baby's tongue-tie status. In Brazil, there is a mandatory frenum inspection law, similar to the newborn screening laws we have for genetic diseases. Perhaps our country needs similar legislation. Some hospitals (and clinics) in the United States have gag orders banning anyone from mentioning tongue-ties to parents (by threat of termination). These rules are scientifically and ethically unacceptable and should be abolished. Tongue-ties are real and they can cause serious harm to babies, children, and adults.

If a baby is assessed in the hospital, and he has an obvious to-the-tip tie, informing the parents of the presence of the tie is critical. It should not be snipped before the parents are informed (this does happen!), and the parents should be educated about the issues that can potentially arise in the future. Ideally, someone trained in tongue-tie release should be the one to perform the frenotomy or frenectomy. The procedure is not complicated, but if the provider performing the procedure has not been properly trained, more injury than benefit may result—not in a physical way (although it can happen), but more in a psychological way. If the parents think that the baby has been treated, but the release was incomplete, they may not seek help for nursing issues that arise afterward. This delay in treatment can be just as detrimental to the health of the baby and mother as if the tongue tie was never diagnosed. How should the procedure and assessment be performed?

The first person to recognize that a child is struggling should refer the parents to a therapist to try nonsurgical intervention first. For babies, this person is the lactation consultant, who will be the quarterback of the team and refer out for care. This lactation consultant should have up-to-date knowledge of tongue-ties, lip-ties, and their impact on function. Then the lactation consultant should refer to a specialist if a tie is suspected. Tongue-tie release should be performed by a knowledgeable and experienced tongue-tie provider, either in the hospital or in the community.

It should go without saying that proper infection control procedures, such as wearing gloves, a mask, and washing hands, are critical, but as some popular videos on YouTube for tongue-tie release show—many clinicians think it's so easy it can be done without gloves on, without a light source, and without proper positioning or swaddling to reduce movement of the baby. Just get in, get out, and on to the next patient. So, if this isn't the correct way to go about the procedure, what are the best practices to follow? Begin by taking a full history of the birth, any complications associated with it, the vitamin K status and any hospital interventions or procedures already performed. Discuss the child's symptoms, including poor latch, gassiness, spitting up, frustration at breast or bottle, clicking or smacking noises, and other issues that can be discovered from the intake questionnaire (located in the Appendix). Discuss the mother's symptoms, such as bleeding, blistered or cracked nipples, amount of pain, poor breast drainage, mastitis, plugged ducts, engorgement, and if one breast hurts more than the other. Combine all of these factors to create a clinical picture of the functional issues that a tongue-tie may be causing. If a baby does not have any symptoms, and a mother does not have any symptoms, then there is no tongue-tie from a functional standpoint, and no treatment is necessary. What number of check marks on the form indicates a tongue-tie is present? If the number is higher than the square root of 42 multiplied by 8 factorial and if the moon is at its farthest orbit from the earth, then it is a tongue-tie...just kidding. There is no "magic number" or formula to follow, because these are real people with real problems, and it is a clinical picture that must be married to the anatomical findings on the clinical exam—in other words, it requires a combination of both art and science. In real life, it is difficult to use numbering systems. What if mom's pain is a 10/10, but the decision tree says "no" or "maybe" based on appearance or function? In these situations, if releasing the posterior tongue-tie causes the pain to resolve immediately, the mother is forever grateful that she wasn't sent away because her baby only scored a 12 instead of a 15 (just hypothetical, no particular assessment in mind).

Exam

For the clinical exam, the baby should be on an exam table, a lap board in the knee-to-knee position, or a dentist's chair. First, check the tightness or flexibility of the lips, feeling for a maxillary lip-tie or buccal-ties in the upper cheeks especially. Then lift the lip. If the papilla blanches or turns white, if the child is in distress when lifting, or if there is a crease on the outside of the upper lip or it doesn't evert normally, then it is likely a lip-tie. When checking under the tongue, if there is a membrane that is restrictive, tight, thick, or too short, then there is a tie in the presence of the defining symptoms. Run a finger back and forth underneath the tongue to check for tightness submucosally—a posterior tongue-tie. Lift up on the tongue with two index fingers when coming from behind, and the tie will pop up if present.

Treatment

Treatment should be performed in the office or the hospital, with no sedation and no general anesthesia. There are almost no circumstances that justify sedation or general anesthesia in a baby less than 12 months old for this procedure because there are capable providers willing and able to perform it safely and effectively in office with no sedation. If scissors are used, multiple cuts must be made to release the entire restriction and not just the sail of the frenum. Cuts must be made while visualizing the area with proper illumination. Further, proper infection control (gloves) and proper restraint of the baby (in either a swaddle, blanket, or with assistants holding the head and body) must be practiced. If a laser is used, all laser safety protocols must be strictly followed, including protective eyewear for the baby. The baby should be put to breast as soon as possible after the procedure, in a private nursing area. Providers should give adequate postoperative instructions, including proper wound care stretches and exercises to be performed. These exercises should be for a duration of at least 2 weeks and at least 3 or 4 times a day at a minimum. The biggest risk of the procedure is that the wound heals back together and needs to be re-treated. Stretching and having parents put on gloves before leaving and coaching them through the motion can help reduce this complication. A 1-week follow-up with the provider should be scheduled to ensure healing is progressing well and no reattachment is occuring. Parents should be counseled to return to the provider's office for additional follow-ups if symptoms return. The lactation consultant should be seen within 24 hours ideally, with follow-up visits scheduled as needed. Any other consults, such as a bodyworker, chiropractor, or craniosacral therapist, should be recommended by the provider or lactation consultant as needed.

Toddlers and Preschool-Age Children

The recommendations for babies carry over well for this age group. They should begin with an evaluation of speech or feeding by a specialist, such as a speech-language pathologist or occupational therapist. After an evaluation and unsuccessful therapy or identification of a restriction, a referral to a provider who has a history of successfully releasing tethered oral tissues and who has the latest knowledge and training should be made. This provider should have a questionnaire for the parent to help determine the primary, secondary, and tertiary issues that could be affecting the child due to the tongue-tie (see Appendix).

After the survey, a thorough examination should be performed. Protrusion or sticking out the tongue is not an appropriate measure to determine if a child or baby has a tongue-tie. Lay the child in a dentist's chair or on an exam table, look at the mouth while positioned behind the head, and use a light to examine the mouth wide open. If you cannot get inside the mouth, then refer to someone who can—likely a pediatric dentist because they have special tools, such as mouth props and bite blocks, to get into the mouth when children don't want to open, and that's what they do all day, every day. The child should be able to elevate the tongue almost to the palate (or you should be able to lift the tongue and see whether it is able to lift or not). The child should be able to move the tongue to clean all of the teeth. The tongue should be able to stick out halfway down the chin or more, but some children who can do this still have restrictions.

Treatment

It is tempting to treat this age group under general anesthesia or sedation. If they are already having another procedure, such as a tonsillectomy, performing the procedure at the same time makes sense. However, for a frenectomy alone, it is better for the child, parent, and the healthcare system to perform the procedure in the office. With a CO_2 laser, it takes about 10 seconds to safely and fully release the tongue. A lip-tie typically takes 15 to 20 seconds. Laser safety glasses are required, and having enough assistance to prevent untoward movement during the procedure is key. Ideally, parents should not be asked to restrain the child unless there is no other option. Parents who wish to participate may hold the hands of younger patients, but often they are in a different room or sit in a chair in the same room. Exercises and stretching protocols along with postoperative instructions are provided to the parents. Working with a myofunctional therapist both before and after the release can help retrain the tongue muscles and ensure proper function for the child.

School-Age Children and Adolescents

Much like toddlers, school-age children and adolescents should first try therapy for speech or feeding issues. If therapy fails or is not progressing and a tie is suspected, a referral to a tie-savvy practitioner is a good next step. After a questionnaire and examination, the most common finding is a posterior tongue-tie. Classic to-the-tip tongue-ties are more often identified at birth or in early childhood; however, to-the-tip ties can be found in adolescents as well. The procedure is performed in the office in this age group, and often only local anesthetic (topical and injected) is all that is required. Some very anxious older children or teens may need an oral anxiolytic. Normally nitrous oxide, or laughing gas, works well for mild-to-moderate anxiety, but some may need something stronger. A full release is key, and myofunctional therapy before and after the release is the best way to ensure successful retraining of the tongue. Normally the wound is left open to heal by secondary intention, but if the child will not be compliant with exercises or the wound stretching protocol, consider placing resorbable chromic gut sutures to close the wound. If no exercises are performed, a wound closed with sutures will heal better than a wound left open, but if exercises can be performed, then leaving the wound open is the best option.

Adults

Adults often have struggled their entire life with feeding, swallowing, speech, neck tension, shoulder pain, forward-head posture, narrow palate, and headaches. Most don't realize they have a tongue-tie until their child is diagnosed with one, and the provider mentions that it can be genetic. Often one or both parents will realize they, too, have a tongue-tie and fit the symptoms and request a release. Adults are much more complicated than children and have years of baggage and medical sequelae from decades of abnormal function. Adults are best managed by a general dentist, an oral surgeon, or ENT who knows the structures of the mouth intimately, and can more effectively manage complex adult medical issues than a pediatric dentist or pediatrician.

For adults, myofunctional therapy should be started before the release and continue afterward, using an individualized plan that is supervised by the therapist. If the diamond-shaped wound is left open to heal, it should be stressed that stretching it open and ensuring that it is open, especially in the morning, is key to preventing reattachment and the return of symptoms. Normally the release should only involve the mucosa and connective tissue (fascia), as in babies and children to release tension. Some surgeons advocate for a deeper release and remove parts of the genioglossus muscle as well. Anytime the muscle is cut, the postoperative pain goes from a 3/10 to a 9/10 or more. It can cause difficulty swallowing and excruciating pain when muscle is released. It can also cause nerve damage, neuralgia, or paresthesia (numbness) of the tongue, and the risk of surgical complications increases greatly. Don't go deep unless it is truly needed and you have the skill to ameliorate any complication with nerves or blood vessels. For most people, a more superficial release of mucosa and fascia is enough to accomplish symptom relief and achieve a functional result.

These best practices will undoubtedly change over time as new research becomes available, but they are a starting point from which to move toward consensus, as this relatively new discipline regarding a congenital disability with an ancient history evolves. More importantly, the ability to prevent and treat the disabilities that arise from abnormal forces in the mouth promises improved quality of life for a large cohort of people.

CHAPTER 29

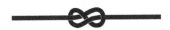

Case Studies

The following case studies detail some of our patients' stories of tongue-ties.

Case 1

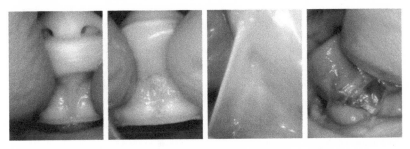

Before and immediately after lip-tie and tongue-tie release.

A baby boy born at 6 lb 14 oz came to our office at 3 weeks old weighing only 7 lb 5 oz. The mother asked the pediatrician if there was a tongue-tie, to which the pediatrician responded that there was no tongue-tie. The mother came to us after a friend suggested she have her baby evaluated. She told us that the pain was a 9 out of 10 every time she nursed her baby. She had begun using a silicone nipple shield, which decreased the pain somewhat, but she was still very uncomfortable. The baby had a poor latch, would fall asleep and slide off the nipple while nursing, and made clicking noises when nursing or taking the bottle. Mom reported that the baby had reflux and was frequently spitting up a large volume of milk. He was tested for pyloric stenosis with an ultrasound, but the test was normal. The baby was also gumming or biting the nipple, couldn't hold a pacifier in his mouth, and was waking up congested and breathing heavily. All of these factors led to mom feeling like it was a full-time job to feed her baby. Meanwhile, the mother had developed creased, flattened, and lipstick-shaped nipples with severe pain when nursing without the shield, and she was told by her doctor that it was normal to have painful nipples.

5. Has your infant experienced any of the following?
- ✓ Poor latch
- ✓ Falls asleep while attempting to nurse
- ✓ Slides off the nipple when attempting to latch
- ___ Colic symptoms
- ✓ Reflux symptoms
- ✓ Clicking noises when nursing or taking bottle
- ✓ Spits up often — *thrown it all up*
- ___ Gassy / Fussy often
- ___ Poor weight gain *(Good wt. gain)*

- ___ Gumming or chewing your nipple when nursing
- ✓ Unable to hold a pacifier in his or her mouth
- ___ Short sleeping requiring feedings every 1-2hrs
- ✓ Snoring, heavy breathing or any sleep apnea
- ✓ Feels like a full time job just to feed baby
- ✓ Waking up congested

Other: _Currently using nipple shield_

6. Is your infant taking any medications? ___ Reflux ___ Thrush Name of medication: _N/A_

7. Has your infant had a prior surgery to correct the tongue or lip tie? If yes, when and where?
_No_

7. Do you have any of the following signs or symptoms?
- ___ Creased, flattened or blanched nipples
- ___ Blistered or cut nipples
- ___ Bleeding nipples
- ___ Severe pain when your infant attempts to latch *(mild)* *on/no pain*
- ✓ Mild pain when your infant latches

- ___ Poor or incomplete breast drainage
- ___ Infected nipples or breasts
- ___ Plugged ducts or mastitis
- ___ Nipple thrush
- ___ None of the above

Unfortunately, this story is repeated daily in offices around the country (and world) that care for babies and mothers with nursing difficulties. Often the problems are caused by undiagnosed tongue-ties and misinformed or uninformed providers. This story could be the same as those of many mothers reading this book, and it is likely one that has been encountered by most of the providers reading this book. Too often, these babies will be given reflux medications like Zantac®, and because they are not gaining weight, they will be given formula. This mother claimed she wasn't told her baby had any issues with weight gain.

This baby's tongue and lip were released, and immediately after the procedure, he was nursed. His mother reported that nursing was more comfortable, with a deeper latch. The clicking noises were gone. The only explanation for this result was that the tongue- and lip-tie releases made a difference. The baby was seen for a follow-up visit 2 weeks later. He weighed 9 lbs 5 oz, having gained 32 ounces in 2 weeks, compared with gaining only 7 ounces the first three weeks! Mom told us that she no longer needed a nipple shield and her milk supply had doubled! Often mothers think that supply issues are their "fault," but it is actually a supply and demand issue. If the baby cannot draw the milk out, the body will not respond and make more milk.

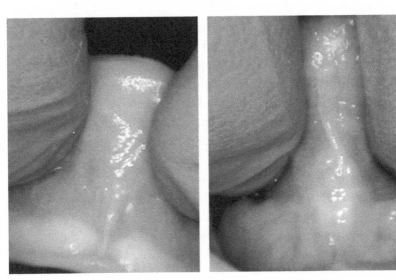

Lip- and tongue-tie release healing, two weeks following the procedure

These results—increased weight gain, less pain, increased milk supply, and less spitting up—are a frequent occurrence in offices where tongue-tie releases are competently performed. The procedure is performed without general anesthesia or sedation, there is little to no risk, and there are great rewards for mothers and their babies.

Case 2

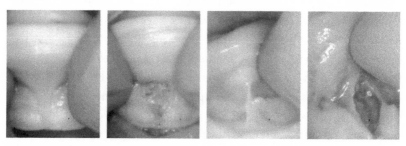

Before and immediately after lip-tie release and tongue-tie release.

This baby boy was clipped in the hospital by a pediatrician, but instead of cutting the frenum, the doctor cut into the body of the tongue above the frenum. Not surprisingly, nursing did not improve after this failed clip. He presented at 6 weeks of age and was eating constantly. He was very fussy, never satisfied or full, took a full hour to feed and caused significant pain for his mother, who therefore required a silicone nursing shield. Immediately after the release, there was significantly decreased pain for the mother, who was able to stop using the shield, and the baby was less fussy and gassy, and ate at a normal rate.

Often, even after a clip or snip into the frenum, nursing issues don't resolve, and the mother still reports pain and trouble feeding. As we've stated before, the clip must be deep enough (often multiple smaller cuts instead of one big snip) and exercises/postoperative stretches must be enacted to prevent reattachment.

Case 3

An almost three-week-old male born at 6 lb 6 oz with a history of laryngomalacia presented at a weight of 6 lb 9 oz. He had poor weight gain and difficulty nursing. He vomited most of his milk after each feeding and he fed inefficiently, so he burned too many calories while feeding and then spit up almost all of what he took in each time. He was very gassy and swallowed air during each nursing session. He was fussy from being hungry all the time and from the gas in his belly. He had seen an ENT for laryngomalacia, and the pediatrician, ENT, and other providers thought he was not gaining weight for that reason. Mom had developed creased, flattened, blistered, and bleeding nipples, with 6 out of 10 pain. The IBCLC referred the baby for an evaluation, and he was found to have a posterior, restrictive tongue-tie and a Kotlow Class 3 lip-tie extending to the ridge. Just those two tiny strings were causing huge issues for this baby.

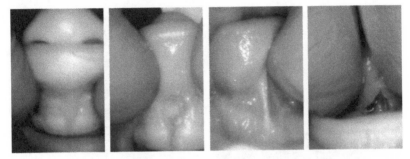

Before and immediately after lip-tie release, and tongue-tie release.

The upper lip and posterior tongue ties were vaporized by the CO_2 laser, a diamond shape was achieved under each site, and the mother immediately noticed a different latch that was deeper and much less painful. Her baby stopped spitting up his milk, and she was overjoyed. One week later, she went to an ENT to evaluate his laryngomalacia because the ENT wanted to do surgery if he was not gaining weight. At this visit, one week after his release, he weighed 7 lb 2 oz, a 9-ounce gain in just one week. This baby had not gained hardly any weight for the first three weeks of his life, but now he was gaining faster than normal—just from having his posterior tongue- and lip-ties released. Neither restriction had been recognized during previous examinations at other offices. A week after his ENT visit, and two weeks after the release, his weight was up to 7 lb 14.5 oz—a difference of 12.5 ounces over the past 7 days, and 21.5 ounces in 2 weeks. Mom reported that before his release, he could take only 2 oz and he spat up most of it. Two weeks post-release, he could take 4 oz per feeding and didn't spit up any at all. He was able to avoid invasive surgery and general anesthesia because he was doing so much better and gaining weight from a 15-second in-office procedure.

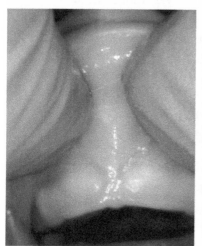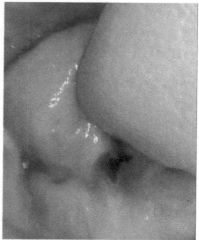

2-week follow-up of lip and tongue

A year later, this child returned for a dental cleaning at our office. His mother stated that he had achieved a normal growth curve, his laryngomalacia had resolved, and he had nursed well for a year. On examination at that visit, he had normal mobility of his tongue and lip, and his mother indicated her profound gratitude for his progress.

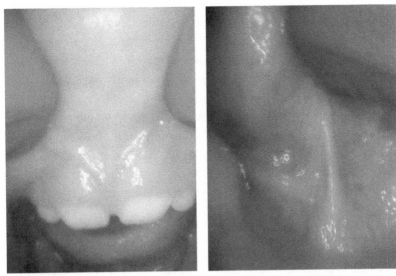

1-year follow-up of lip and tongue. Notice that frena are still present, but are less restrictive and tight.

Case 4

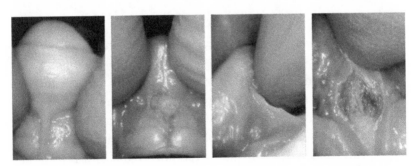

Before and immediately after lip-tie release and tongue-tie release.

This three-week-old male weighed 7 lb 10 oz at birth and now weighed 7 lb 3.5 oz. He was already clipped at the local hospital on day 3 after struggling with nursing and being diagnosed with a tie. Mom did not notice any difference in breastfeeding after the clip. A 1-mm nick had been made in the frenum, and a large amount of restrictive tissue still remained. It is very common to see babies who require more complete releases after initial treatment. In this case, the mother was triple feeding the baby, but he had not regained his birth weight at 3 weeks despite tremendous effort from mom. He made clicking noises while feeding and mom was in significant pain every time he nursed.

After the release, we achieved a diamond shape on both the lip and tongue for a full release, and mom reported no pain at all when nursing. He nursed for a much shorter time and actually took 9 oz during the weighted feed right after the procedure in our office. Mom noticed dramatically better milk transfer.

Case 5

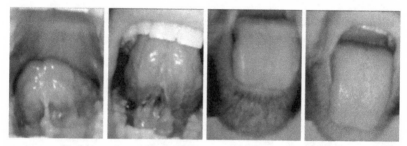

Before and immediately after elevation and protrusion.

This 36-year-old male had a history of tongue-tie at birth and had been clipped in the hospital. As we've seen, clips may not do much if performed incompletely. Many people think that children "grow out of" tongue-ties or that the strings stretch with time. As this case clearly shows, this tongue-tie did not stretch. If it is restricted in infancy, or snipped incompletely early on, it will remain that way until it is released properly. This man had difficulty speaking fast and tired easily when speaking, so he learned to use short sentences. He also mumbled or spoke quietly when speaking.

Immediately after his release, it was easier for him to talk, he didn't get tired when speaking, and he had greatly improved mobility. He also had malocclusion, with the lower incisors being pulled inward, as illustrated in the photo. It is impossible to clean your teeth properly with this degree of restriction.

Case 6

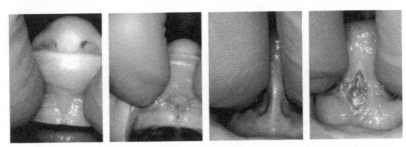

Before and immediately after lip-tie release and tongue-tie release.

A four-day-old male presented with a shallow latch, reflux, colic, snoring, heavy breathing, short sleeping (waking every 1 to 2 hours), sliding off the nipple while attempting to latch, and producing a clicking or smacking noise when nursing. Mom had developed creased, flattened, bleeding, and blistered nipples, severe pain when nursing, infected, plugged ducts, and recent-onset mastitis. The pediatrician said there was "nothing wrong" and "no tongue-tie" when the mother inquired about a possible tongue-tie. The mother is a speech therapist and therefore referred herself. This baby had a tight upper lip-tie and a restrictive posterior or submucosal tongue-tie.

Immediately after the procedure, while they were still in our office, the new mother observed resolution of the baby's symptoms. She was unable to nurse due to severe pain from the mastitis, but the baby had a deeper latch on the bottle, made no clicking noises, didn't fuss while eating, didn't spit up, and took the whole 4-oz bottle in 10 minutes. Previous feedings lasted 60 minutes.

Case 7

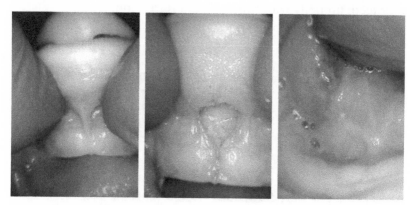

Before and immediately after lip-tie release, normal tongue.

This baby had only a lip-tie and no tongue-tie. There was no speed bump feel when sweeping the finger under the tongue; she had good elevation and no issues with cupping the tongue. Her lip was restricted, blanched when lifted and was painful when lifted. Her lip curled under when she nursed. Her lip-tie caused her to regurgitate and be gassy, and fussy. Her mother reported a poor, shallow latch, painful nursing, distorted nipple shape, and she had to use a silicone nipple shield to nurse her.

Immediately after the release, her issues disappeared. The baby could latch better and the mother could nurse more comfortably, with no nipple shield needed. The infant gained 17 ounces over the following 7 days. Normal weight gain would have been around 7 ounces. Her 1-week follow-up sheet is below. Not every low frenum is a lip-tie, but if it is restricted and the baby and mother have symptoms, then a tie-savvy provider should evaluate it. A simple 15-second procedure with virtually no risk saved this nursing relationship and alleviated the mother's pain as well as the baby's.

Birth weight 6 lb 13oz Weight at initial visit 8 lb 6oz Weight today 9 lb 7

Did you continue to stretch the surgical sites well each day? ✓ yes ___ no

Did you have follow up with your lactation consultant? ✓ yes ___ no ___ N/A

1. Have you noticed any difference in your baby's latch? Any improvement in other symptoms like gassiness, fussiness, reflux, choking, milk dribbling out, spitting up, sleeping better, holding a pacifier better, no clicking noise, etc.?

   yes, latching better, gassiness, fussiness, spitting up all improved

2. Have you noticed any differences for you? If baby is not breastfeeding please write N/A. (more comfortable, less pain, increased supply, normal nipple shape, no nipple shield needed etc.)

3. Anything else you have noticed since the surgery?

   no

4. Additional comments concerning your experience at our office or with the surgery?

   great experience, would recommend highly

Dr. Notes: didn't even need tongue   gained one pound since

Notice differen right off bat. procedure

Thank you,

Case 8

A 3-year 4-month-old girl suffered from speech, feeding, and sleep issues. As an infant, she had difficulty nursing, and her mother had to abandon nursing and use formula. However, even formula proved to be a struggle, and mom had to use thickener and a special nipple to feed her. She had a modified barium swallow test at 6 months old, and she struggled with swallowing the first 2 years of her life. At the time of her visit, at age 3, she choked on foods, had a hard time finishing meals, grazed on food all day, had trouble feeding herself, spit out food, ate slowly, and it was a "daily fight" to nourish her, according to her mother. When she spoke, she had a hard time speaking fast, and she sometimes stuttered. Her sleep was another major issue. She kicked and moved around a lot at night, woke up tired and not refreshed, slept with her mouth open, snored, and even gasped for air when sleeping. She also mouth breathed during the day and suffered from constipation (likely from poorly chewed and therefore poorly digested food).

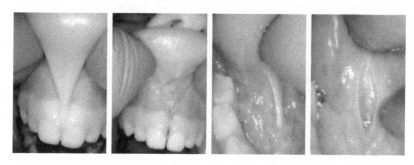

Before and immediately after lip-tie release and tongue-tie release.

On examination, this little girl had a lip-tie that was restricting the mobility of her upper lip and was blanching the tissue when lifted, although her teeth were together with no gap. In addition, she had a restrictive posterior tongue-tie that was not obvious on first inspection, but could be observed when the tongue was elevated with two fingers. The latter was tight and limited both mobility and function. The release was uneventful, with no need for sedation, nitrous oxide or general anesthesia, and after about 15 seconds of lasing for the lip-tie and about 10 seconds for the tongue-tie, it was complete. The only anesthetic used was topical compounded lidocaine, prilocaine, and tetracaine jelly. She cried for a minute or so, and then calmed down quickly. That night, mom noticed a difference in speech, and it was easier for the patient to eat and swallow. She also slept much more deeply and peacefully. At the 1-week follow-up, her mother reported that she was speaking more and more clearly, appeared increasingly confident when feeding herself, and no longer choked on foods, which occurred daily before. She ate eggs and hamburger, which she had been unable to tolerate before. Her sleep was much improved, with less movement, snoring, and mouth breathing. Her mother observed that she drooled more than before, but this subsided around the third week. Mother and child continued stretches in addition to myofunctional exercises for 3 weeks.

This case illustrates that infants who suffer from poor swallowing and reflux and need thickener for their bottles should be assessed for posterior tongue and lip-ties. It is much easier and less expensive to correct these abnormalities than for these babies to grow up and struggle with speech, feeding, and sleep quality. A tongue- or lip-tie release addresses the cause of the issue instead of focusing on symptomatic relief. The most consistent and rapid benefit seen after a tongue-tie release in this age group (1 to 4 years) is better-quality sleep leading to better mood and energy. The feeding often improves quickly but therapy is required for full resolution of the swallowing issues. Speech often improves the first week, but again the greatest benefits are realized after additional time and therapy.

Case 9

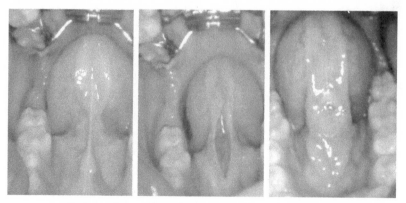

Before release, after release, and one-week follow-up.

This 12-year 7-month-old boy was a dental patient who had been diagnosed with ADHD, anxiety, and some developmental delays, although he was very intelligent and witty. He didn't have much trouble with his speech, but he had already been in therapy for 4 years. He had a history of reflux as a baby and still suffered from reflux 12 years later. His adenoids and tonsils were removed when he was a young child. He complained of neck and shoulder pain daily, was a mouth breather, had frequent constipation, and constantly popped his knuckles and other joints. He was very picky with textures such as meat, cooked vegetables, mashed potatoes, and milk. He would spit out food and instantly vomit if it was not the right texture. He had several sleep issues, including sleeping in strange positions, grinding his teeth and mouth breathing at night, and snoring. He had severe dental crowding and had a palatal expander placed.

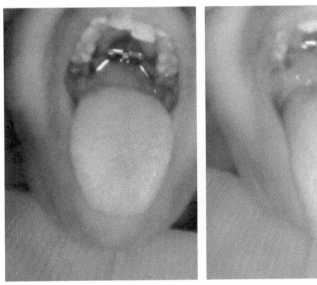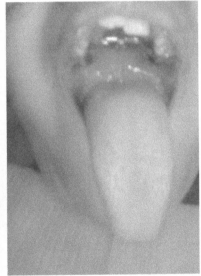

Tongue protrusion before and after release. His protrusion beforehand was within the normal range, but his impaired elevation, coupled with his symptomatic history, made him a candidate for a release.

Upon examination, his tongue-tie was posterior and, at first glance, the frenum appeared totally normal. However, with the symptoms he had, a detailed investigation was appropriate. Upon digital exam, the submucosal portion of the frenum felt tighter and more restrictive than normal. He could stick his tongue out about halfway down his chin, which is within the normal range, but he had many symptoms that suggested his restriction was causing a problem. Mom was informed a release would likely help with some of his texture symptoms at least, although it was not a guarantee. Mom chose to proceed with treatment, which was uneventful and performed in the office with the CO_2 laser, nitrous oxide, and lidocaine.

At the follow-up visit, the mother remarked that the procedure was very helpful for his feeding and sleep. After the release, she noticed he went to sleep, remained asleep and woke up more refreshed than he did previously. Before the surgery, he woke up at least once every night to go get something to eat. His feeding improved dramatically and he no longer had aversions to textures or vegetables. He even asked for vegetables on a sandwich, which he had never previously done. He stopped grazing on foods, finished his meals, stopped packing his cheeks, and was more relaxed when eating, indicating he could swallow more easily. In addition, he stopped popping his knuckles, neck, and other joints as frequently and stopped complaining of shoulder pain. He remarked it was "easier to move [his] neck." He hadn't had a headache, which would normally occur a few times a week; his improved chewing (and therefore more complete digestion) alleviated his constipation. This boy's quality of life was greatly affected by the release of a seemingly normal frenum that was, in his case, functionally too tight.

Case 10

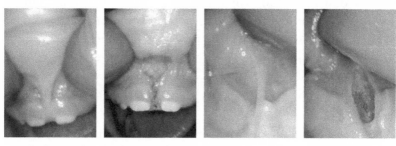

Before and immediately after lip-tie release, and tongue-tie release.

This 10-month-old boy was referred by a speech therapist for a tongue- and lip-tie evaluation. He and his mother struggled valiantly to nurse, but they had to abandon breastfeeding at 1 month due to his poor latch, colic, reflux, and gassiness. Mom was triple feeding (nursing, pumping, and feeding the expressed breast milk), and he still had a hard time gaining weight. His lip curled under when nursing, and he was taking an hour for each feeding. He had reflux and was medicated with ranitidine (Zantac®), with little improvement. He had recurrent ear infections necessitating ear tubes. These issues, unfortunately, did not improve when switching to a bottle, and he still struggled even taking a bottle. His mother was the only one who could feed him, and when he went to daycare, he would only take an ounce or two the whole day, because he was so frustrated and couldn't even take the bottle. He slept poorly and awakened up to 3 to 4 times per night, every night, for 10 months. His parents were exhausted and drained, emotionally and physically. He was examined and diagnosed with a Kotlow Class 4 lip-tie, and a submucosal Kotlow Class 1 posterior tongue-tie. The frenum was not very visible, but it was restricting tongue elevation and normal mobility for this child.

After the 15-second procedure for the lip and 10-second procedure for the tongue, he was quickly soothed and immediately took his bottle faster and without fussing. That first night, he slept through the night without waking up once. He continued to sleep through the night every night, which was life-changing for his parents. He began to finish his whole bottle at daycare, whereas previously he could only take one-fourth of the bottle. He started swallowing solid foods more easily. He exhibited increased babbling, and he even said a new word just after the one-week follow-up: "dada."

Function and symptoms are more important than the appearance.

These are not the "best" cases by any means, but these stories are repeated daily in many offices around the world. Each one could be made into a case study highlighting the impact that removing a tiny string can make on a child's—or even an adult's—life.

CHAPTER 30

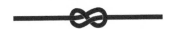

Next Steps For Professionals

I f you'd like to learn more about tongue-ties, there are a number of resources available. Websites, online classes and many references, including scientific journal articles, are listed in the next few pages. There are quite a few research publications available about nursing, fewer on speech, smaller numbers on feeding, and almost none on adults with other concurrent issues and tongue-ties. The field is ripe for research by anyone with a desire to increase our collective knowledge in this area.

This book is a humble attempt to provide the most up-to-date and latest thinking in this field, but most of the ideas presented in this book may eventually be shown to be incomplete, as evidence-based care is an ever-evolving paradigm. However, that's the way we humans move forward. As Charles Sidney Burwell, past dean of the Harvard Medical School, famously said, "Half of what we are going to teach you is wrong, and half of it is right. Our problem is that we don't know which half is which." Now that we understand the many functional abnormalities a tongue-tie can cause, it's clear that children and adults with difficulties of speech, eating and sleep deserve to be evaluated by people skilled in the disciplines described here.

Tongue-ties have profound effects on the quality of life families are able to enjoy during many critical stages of development of the children they affect. Both parents and children are impacted by the dysfunction experienced by those who have tongue- or lip-ties. Releasing the ties can relieve many more stressors than most people realize are part of the syndrome of tethered oral tissues. For further education about the issues these parents and patients face, here are some recommended courses and resources. This is not an endorsement of everything written on the websites or said in the courses, but they are a good place to start. Thank you for joining us on this journey. We are grateful for this opportunity to give a voice to these patients and families, many of whom have struggled for years, waiting for their stories to be told. Let's pursue more research, education, and knowledge together in this evolving field, and encourage other patients, parents, and providers to learn more about how best to help those with tethered oral tissues.

Resources

Tongue-Tied Academy, an online comprehensive course that helps you identify and treat tongue and lip ties with confidence can be found at: www.TongueTiedAcademy.com

On the Alabama Tongue-Tie Center website, you can browse our video library, download all of our patient forms and a list of materials we use in our office. Please visit: www.TongueTieAL.com/Professionals

To order bulk copies of *Tongue-Tied*, please visit www.TongueTieAL.com/Book

Tongue-Tied is available in an audiobook version as well on Audible and Amazon.

Other Selected Resources for Professionals

TOTS (Tethered Oral Tissues Specialty) Training Course by Autumn R. Henning, MS, CCC-SLP, COM
http://www.chrysalisfeeding.com

IBCLC Master Class: Oral Rehabilitation of the Breastfeeding Dyad Course https://iparentllc.wixsite.com/ibclcmasterclass

Cranial Nerve Dysfunction and Oral Restrictions in the Precrawling Infant: A Multidisciplinary Class for TOTs

Professionals by Michelle Emanuel, OTR/L
http://www.TummyTimeMethod.com

The Breathe Institute hosts several outstanding, evidence-based courses including The Breathe Course with Dr. Soroush Zaghi and The Breathe Baby course with Dr. Chelsea Pinto focusing on multidisciplinary treatment of adults, and babies respectively. http://www.TheBreatheInstitute.com

GOLD Online Learning has almost 30 courses about tongue-ties from many different speakers and different angles. There are courses for pediatricians, lactation consultants, dentists, and more relating to tongue-tie. https://www.goldlearning.com

Drs. Kaplan and Convissar along with Alison Hazelbaker, PhD, IBCLC, and Peter Vitruk, PhD, authored a *Color Atlas of Infant Tongue-Tie and Lip-Tie Laser Frenectomy*, which is the first textbook written on the subject of laser use for tongue-tie release. https://www.laserfrenectomybook.com

Tongue-Tie Morphogenesis, Impact, Assessment and Treatment by Allison Hazelbaker, PhD, IBCLC, CST, RCST, is a helpful resource detailing the history of tongue-tie and its impact primarily on nursing babies. It also discusses her validated assessment protocol, the HATLFF. http://www.alisonhazelbaker.com/tongue-tie-book/

Tongue-Tie—From Confusion to Clarity by Carmen Fernando, a speech pathologist, is available as an eBook and a paperback that discusses feeding and speech issues related to tongue-tie, as well as history and assessment. https://tonguetie.net/the-book/

Dr. Larry Kotlow is a tongue-tie pioneer who has developed many helpful handouts from courses and scientific articles. These can be found at http://www.kiddsteeth.com. His recent book, *SOS 4 TOTS*, is a helpful resource focusing on babies with tethered oral tissues and the struggles mothers endure to have them treated.

Locate or join the multidisciplinary TOTs Bodywork team www. AnkyloglossiaBodyworkers.com, which includes various research and manual therapy information for parents. You can find someone local to you in the professional directory included on the website.

Dr. Bobby Ghaheri's blog and Facebook page are updated regularly with helpful information. http://www.drghaheri.com/blog/

www.Talktools.com offers Oral-Placement Therapy (OPT) techniques, training, and tools to clients, therapists and parents. Their therapy techniques add a tactile component to feeding and speech therapy, enabling clients to "feel" the movements necessary for the development of speech clarity.

Professional Organizations Relating to Tongue-Ties

IATP (International Affiliation of Tongue-Tie Professionals) https://tonguetieprofessionals.org/

ICAP (International Consortium of Oral Ankylofrenula Professionals) http://www.icapprofessionals.com/

ALSC (American Laser Study Club) http://www.americanlaserstudyclub.org

Myofunctional Therapy Resources

The International Association of Orofacial Myology (IAOM) http://iaom.com

The Academy of Myofunctional Therapy (AOMT) https://aomtinfo.org

The Applied Academy of Myofunctional Sciences (AAMS) https://aamsinfo.org/

The Coulson Institute
https://coulsoninstitute.com/

The Graduate School of Behavioral Health Sciences
https://www.bp.edu/

Resources for Parents

Dr. Baxter's website www.TongueTieAL.com and blog are up-to-date resources for parents and professionals wanting to learn more about tongue-ties. www.TongueTieAL.com/Blog

Dr. Bobby Ghaheri's blog and Facebook page are great resources for learning more. http://www.drghaheri.com/blog/ https://www.facebook.com/DrGhaheriMD/

Facebook groups:

Tongue Tie Babies Support Group
Tongue Tie Lip Tie Baby Support Group
Tongue Tie Kids
Tongue Tied Adults Support Group
Location-specific groups (States, and Regions)

"Preferred-Provider List"
https://www.tt-lt-support-network.com/

www.AnkyloglossiaBodyworkers.com is a source for information, research and provider directory specifically for bodyworkers evaluating and treating babies with TOTs.

www.TummyTimeMethod.com is a source for tummy time education and support, includes provider directory.

www.Pathways.org is a source of free developmental information for parents and professionals.

References

1. Marasco L. Letter to the editor regarding N. Sethi, et al., benefits of frenulotomy in infants with ankyloglossia, IJPO (2013), http://dx.doi.org/10.1016/j.ijporl.2013.02.005. Int J Pediatr Otorhinolaryngol 2014;78(3):572.

2. Hong SJ, Cha BG, Kim YS, Lee SK, Chi JG. Tongue Growth during Prenatal Development in Korean Fetuses and Embryos. J Pathol Transl Med 2015;49(6):497–510.

3. Pompéia LE, Ilinsky RS, Ortolani CLF, Faltin K Júnior. Ankyloglossia and its influence on growth and development of the stomatognathic system. Rev Paul Pediatr 2017;35(2):216–21.

4. Obladen M. Much ado about nothing: two millennia of controversy on tongue-tie. Neonatology 2010;97(2):83–9.

5. Fernando C. Tongue Tie--from Confusion to Clarity: A Guide to the Diagnosis and Treatment of Ankyloglossia. Tandem Publications; 1998.

6. Ip S, Chung M, Raman G, Chew P, Magula N, DeVine D, et al. Breastfeeding and maternal and infant health outcomes in developed countries. Evid Rep Technol Assess 2007;(153):1–186.

7. Stuebe A. The risks of not breastfeeding for mothers and infants. Rev Obstet Gynecol 2009;2(4):222–31.

8. Kramer MS, Kakuma R. Optimal duration of exclusive breastfeeding. Cochrane Database Syst Rev 2012;(8): CD003517.

9. Messner AH, Lalakea ML. Ankyloglossia: controversies in management. Int J Pediatr Otorhinolaryngol 2000;54 (2-3):123–31.

10. Buryk M, Bloom D, Shope T. Efficacy of neonatal release of ankyloglossia: a randomized trial. Pediatrics 2011;128(2):280–8.

11.   Berry J, Griffiths M, Westcott C. A double-blind, randomized, controlled trial of tongue-tie division and its immediate effect on breastfeeding. Breastfeed Med 2012;7(3):189–93.

12.   Geddes DT, Langton DB, Gollow I, Jacobs LA, Hartmann PE, Simmer K. Frenulotomy for breastfeeding infants with ankyloglossia: effect on milk removal and sucking mechanism as imaged by ultrasound. Pediatrics 2008;122(1):e188–94.

13.   O'Callahan C, Macary S, Clemente S. The effects of office-based frenotomy for anterior and posterior ankyloglossia on breastfeeding. Int J Pediatr Otorhinolaryngol 2013;77(5):827–32.

14.   Ghaheri BA, Cole M, Fausel SC, Chuop M, Mace JC. Breastfeeding improvement following tongue-tie and lip-tie release: A prospective cohort study. Laryngoscope 2017;127(5):1217–23.

15.   Ghaheri BA, Cole M, Mace JC. Revision Lingual Frenotomy Improves Patient-Reported Breastfeeding Outcomes: A Prospective Cohort Study. J Hum Lact 2018;890334418775624.

16.   Hogan M, Westcott C, Griffiths M. Randomized, controlled trial of division of tongue-tie in infants with feeding problems. J Paediatr Child Health [Internet] 2005; Available from: http://onlinelibrary.wiley.com/doi/10.1111/j.1440-1754.2005.00604.x/full

17.   Kotlow LA. Oral diagnosis of abnormal frenum attachments in neonates and infants: evaluation and treatment of the maxillary and lingual frenum using the Erbium: YAG laser. J Pediatric Dent Care 2004;10(3):11–4.

18.   Kotlow L. Diagnosis and treatment of ankyloglossia and tied maxillary fraenum in infants using Er:YAG and 1064 diode lasers. Eur Arch Paediatr Dent 2011;12(2):106–12.

19.   Kotlow LA. Ankyloglossia (tongue-tie): a diagnostic and treatment quandary. Quintessence Int 1999;30(4):259–62.

20.   Emond A, Ingram J, Johnson D, Blair P, Whitelaw A, Copeland M, et al. Randomised controlled trial of early frenotomy in breastfed infants with mild-moderate tongue-tie. Arch Dis Child Fetal Neonatal Ed 2014;99(3):F189–95.

21. Smith GCS, Pell JP. Parachute use to prevent death and major trauma related to gravitational challenge: systematic review of randomised controlled trials. BMJ 2003;327(7429):1459–61.

22. Osband YB, Altman RL, Patrick PA, Edwards KS. Breastfeeding education and support services offered to pediatric residents in the US. Acad Pediatr 2011;11(1):75–9.

23. Siegel SA. Aerophagia Induced Reflux in Breastfeeding Infants With Ankyloglossia and Shortened Maxillary Labial Frenula (Tongue and Lip Tie). International Journal of Clinical Pediatrics 2016;5(1):6–8.

24. Coryllos E, Genna CW, Salloum AC, Others. Congenital tongue-tie and its impact on breastfeeding. Breastfeeding: Best for Mother and Baby 2004;1–6.

25. de Castro Martinelli RL, Marchesan IQ, Gusmão RJ, de Castro Rodrigues A, Berretin-Felix G. Histological characteristics of altered human lingual frenulum. International Journal of Pediatrics and Child Health 2014;2:5–9.

26. Pransky SM, Lago D, Hong P. Breastfeeding difficulties and oral cavity anomalies: The influence of posterior ankyloglossia and upper-lip ties. Int J Pediatr Otorhinolaryngol 2015;79(10):1714–7.

27. Kotlow LA. Diagnosing and understanding the maxillary lip-tie (superior labial, the maxillary labial frenum) as it relates to breastfeeding. J Hum Lact 2013;29(4):458–64.

28. Flinck A, Paludan A, Matsson L, Holm AK, Axelsson I. Oral findings in a group of newborn Swedish children. Int J Paediatr Dent 1994;4(2):67–73.

29. Ghaheri B. Lip-Tie vs. Normal Frenum [Internet]. Bobby Ghaheri MD Facebook Blog Post2017 [cited 2018 May 29];Available from: https://www.facebook.com/DrGhaheriMD/photos/a.451553228339392.1073741829.329432813884768/807144299446948/?type=3

30. Santa Maria C, Aby J, Truong MT, Thakur Y, Rea S, Messner A. The Superior Labial Frenulum in Newborns: What Is Normal? Glob Pediatr Health 2017;4:2333794X17718896.

31. Centers for Disease Control and Prevention. Breastfeeding Report Card, 2016. CDC; 2016.

32.   Section on Breastfeeding. Breastfeeding and the use of human milk. Pediatrics 2012;129(3):e827–41.

33.   Odom EC, Li R, Scanlon KS, Perrine CG, Grummer-Strawn L. Reasons for earlier than desired cessation of breastfeeding. Pediatrics 2013;131(3):e726–32.

34.   Hazelbaker AK. The assessment tool for lingual frenulum function (ATLFF): Use in a lactation consultant private practice. 1993;

35.   Srinivasan A, Dobrich C, Mitnick H, Feldman P. Ankyloglossia in breastfeeding infants: the effect of frenotomy on maternal nipple pain and latch. Breastfeed Med 2006;1(4):216–24.

36.   Martinelli RL de C, Marchesan IQ, Berretin-Felix G. Lingual frenulum protocol with scores for infants. Int J Orofacial Myology 2012;38:104–12.

37.   Lopes de Castro Martinelli R, Queiroz Marchesan I, Berretin-Felix G. Protocolo de avaliação do frênulo lingual para bebês: relação entre aspectos anatômicos e funcionais. Revista CEFAC [Internet] 2013;15(3). Available from: http://www.redalyc.org/html/1693/169327929012/

38.   Martinelli RL de C, Marchesan IQ, Lauris JR, Honório HM, Gusmão RJ, Berretin-Felix G. Validade e confiabilidade da triagem: "teste da linguinha." Rev CEFAC 2016;18(6):1323–31.

39.   FDA. FDA review results in new warnings about using general anesthetics and sedation drugs in young children and pregnant women [Internet]. FDA Drug Safety Communications2016 [cited 2018 May 29];Available from: https://www.fda.gov/downloads/Drugs/DrugSafety/UCM533197.pdf

40.   Reddy SV. Effect of general anesthetics on the developing brain. J Anaesthesiol Clin Pharmacol [Internet] 2012;Available from: https://www.ncbi.nlm.nih.gov/pmc/articles/PMC3275974/

41.   Rhoades DR, McFarland KF, Finch WH, Johnson AO. Speaking and interruptions during primary care office visits. Fam Med 2001;33(7):528–32.

42.   Romanos GE, Belikov AV, Skrypnik AV, Feldchtein FI, Smirnov MZ, Altshuler GB. Uncovering dental implants using a new thermo-optically powered (TOP) technology with tissue air-cooling. Lasers Surg Med 2015;47(5):411–20.

43.   Georgios E. Romanos D. Diode Laser Soft-Tissue Surgery: Advancements Aimed at Consistent Cutting, Improved Clinical Outcomes. Compend Contin Educ Dent [Internet] 2013 [cited 2018 Jun 18]; Available from: https://cced.cdeworld. com/courses/20875-Diode_Laser_Soft-Tissue_Surgery:Advancements_Aimed_ at_Consistent_Cutting-Improved_Clinical_Outcomes

44.   Shavit I, Peri-Front Y, Rosen-Walther A, Grunau RE, Neuman G, Nachmani O, et al. A Randomized Trial to Evaluate the Effect of Two Topical Anesthetics on Pain Response During Frenotomy in Young Infants. Pain Med 2017;18(2):356–62.

45.   Ovental A, Marom R, Botzer E, Batscha N, Dollberg S. Using topical benzocaine before lingual frenotomy did not reduce crying and should be discouraged. Acta Paediatr 2014;103(7):780–2.

46.   Shah PS, Herbozo C, Aliwalas LL, Shah VS. Breastfeeding or breast milk for procedural pain in neonates. Cochrane Database Syst Rev 2012;12:CD004950.

47.   Simonse E, Mulder PGH, van Beek RHT. Analgesic effect of breast milk versus sucrose for analgesia during heel lance in late preterm infants. Pediatrics 2012;129(4):657–63.

48.   So T-Y, Farrington E. Topical benzocaine-induced methemoglobinemia in the pediatric population. J Pediatr Health Care 2008;22(6):335–9; quiz 340–1.

49.   Haytac MC, Ozcelik O. Evaluation of patient perceptions after frenectomy operations: a comparison of carbon dioxide laser and scalpel techniques. J Periodontol 2006;77(11):1815–9.

50.   Woolridge MW. The "anatomy" of infant sucking. Midwifery 1986;2(4):164–71.

51.   Elad D, Kozlovsky P, Blum O, Laine AF, Po MJ, Botzer E, et al. Biomechanics of milk extraction during breast-feeding. Proc Natl Acad Sci U S A 2014;111(14):5230–5.

52.   Chu MW, Bloom DC. Posterior ankyloglossia: a case report. Int J Pediatr Otorhinolaryngol 2009;73(6):881–3.

53.   Kotlow LA. The influence of the maxillary frenum on the development and pattern of dental caries on anterior teeth in breastfeeding infants: prevention, diagnosis, and treatment. J Hum Lact 2010;26(3):304–8.

54. Hearnsberger D. Eat-Drink-Be Nourished: Development and Disorder in Pediatric Feeding [Internet]. Available from: https://www.eatdrinkbenourished.com/

55. Hazelbaker A. Lactation Education Resources - Alison Hazelbaker: Online Video Conference [Internet]. [cited 2018 Jun 29];Available from: https://www.lactationtraining.com/our-courses/online-conferences/alison-hazelbaker-conference

56. Gatto K. Understanding the Orofacial Complex: The Evolution of Dysfunction. Outskirts Press; 2016.

57. Bahr D. Nobody Ever Told Me (or my Mother) That!: Everything from Bottles and Breathing to Healthy Speech Development. 1 edition. Sensory World; 2010.

58. Potock M. Personal Communication. 2018.

59. Henning A. Tethered Oral Tissues Specialty Training. 2017.

60. Silva MC, Costa MLVCM da, Nemr K, Marchesan IQ. Lingual frenulum alteration and chewing interference. Rev CEFAC 2009;11:363–9.

61. Baxter R, Hughes L. Speech and Feeding Improvements in Children After Posterior Tongue-Tie Release: A Case Series. International Journal of Clinical Pediatrics [Internet] 2018 [cited 2018 Jun 28];0(0). Available from: http://www.theijcp.org/index.php/ijcp/article/view/295/254

62. Articulation | Definition of articulation in English by Oxford Dictionaries [Internet]. Oxford Dictionaries | English [cited 2018 Jun 29];Available from: https://en.oxforddictionaries.com/definition/articulation

63. Definition of Articulation [Internet]. Merriam-Webster Dictionary [cited 2018 Jun 29];Available from: https://www.merriam-webster.com/dictionary/articulation

64. Yoon AJ, Zaghi S, Ha S, Law CS, Guilleminault C, Liu SY. Ankyloglossia as a risk factor for maxillary hypoplasia and soft palate elongation: A functional - morphological study. Orthod Craniofac Res 2017;20(4):237–44.

65. Messner AH, Lalakea ML. The effect of ankyloglossia on speech in children. Otolaryngol Head Neck Surg 2002;127(6):539–45.

66. Ito Y, Shimizu T, Nakamura T. Effectiveness of tongue-tie division for speech disorder in children. Pediatrics [Internet] 2015;Available from: http://onlinelibrary.wiley.com/doi/10.1111/ped.12474/full

67. Walls A, Pierce M, Wang H, Steehler A, Steehler M, Harley EH Jr. Parental perception of speech and tongue mobility in three-year olds after neonatal frenotomy. Int J Pediatr Otorhinolaryngol 2014;78(1):128–31.

68. Dollberg S, Manor Y, Makai E, Botzer E. Evaluation of speech intelligibility in children with tongue-tie. Acta Pædiatrica [Internet] 2011;Available from: http://onlinelibrary.wiley.com/doi/10.1111/j.1651-2227.2011.02265.x/full

69. Webb AN, Hao W, Hong P. The effect of tongue-tie division on breastfeeding and speech articulation: a systematic review. Int J Pediatr Otorhinolaryngol 2013;77(5):635–46.

70. Chinnadurai S, Francis DO, Epstein RA, Morad A, Kohanim S, McPheeters M. Treatment of ankyloglossia for reasons other than breastfeeding: a systematic review. Pediatrics 2015;135(6):e1467–74.

71. Lalakea ML, Messner AH. Ankyloglossia: the adolescent and adult perspective. Otolaryngol Head Neck Surg 2003;128(5):746–52.

72. Lalakea ML, Messner AH. Ankyloglossia: does it matter? Pediatr Clin North Am 2003;50(2):381–97.

73. Mattar SEM, Anselmo-Lima WT, Valera FCP, Matsumoto MAN. Skeletal and occlusal characteristics in mouth-breathing pre-school children. J Clin Pediatr Dent 2004;28(4):315–8.

74. Harari D, Redlich M, Miri S, Hamud T, Gross M. The effect of mouth breathing versus nasal breathing on dentofacial and craniofacial development in orthodontic patients. Laryngoscope 2010;120(10):2089–93.

75. Yoon A, Zaghi S, Weitzman R, Ha S, Law CS, Guilleminault C, et al. Toward a functional definition of ankyloglossia: validating current grading scales for lingual frenulum length and tongue mobility in 1052 subjects. Sleep Breath 2017;21(3):767–75.

76. Palmer B. The Importance of Breastfeeding As It Relates to Total Health [Internet]. Brian Palmer, DDS For Better Health 2002 [cited 2018 May 29];Available from: http://www.brianpalmerdds.com/pdf/section_A.pdf

77. Lin S. Dental Diet: The Surprising Link Between Your Teeth, Real Food, and Life-Changing Natural Health The. Hay House, Incorporated; 2019.

78. Moss ML, Salentijn L. The primary role of functional matrices in facial growth. Am J Orthod 1969;55(6):566–77.

79. Trabalon M, Schaal B. It takes a mouth to eat and a nose to breathe: abnormal oral respiration affects neonates' oral competence and systemic adaptation. Int J Pediatr 2012;2012:207605.

80. Eltzschig HK, Carmeliet P. Hypoxia and inflammation. N Engl J Med 2011;364(7):656–65.

81. Izuhara Y, Matsumoto H, Nagasaki T, Kanemitsu Y, Murase K, Ito I, et al. Mouth breathing, another risk factor for asthma: the Nagahama Study. Allergy 2016;71(7):1031–6.

82. Yamaguchi H, Tada S, Nakanishi Y, Kawaminami S, Shin T, Tabata R, et al. Association between Mouth Breathing and Atopic Dermatitis in Japanese Children 2-6 years Old: A Population-Based Cross-Sectional Study. PLoS One 2015;10(4):e0125916.

83. Hang WM, Gelb M. Airway Centric® TMJ philosophy/Airway Centric® orthodontics ushers in the post-retraction world of orthodontics. Cranio 2017;35(2):68–78.

84. Huang YS, Quo S, Berkowski JA, Guilleminault C. Short lingual frenulum and obstructive sleep apnea in children. Int J Pediatr Res [Internet] 2015;1(003). Available from: http://orofacialintegrity.com/wp-content/uploads/2015/05/short-ling-frenum-and-sleep-apnea.pdf

85. Palmer B. Otitis Media: An Anatomical Perspective [Internet]. Brian Palmer, DDS For Better Health 2001 [cited 2018 May 29];Available from: http://www.brianpalmerdds.com/pdf/Otitis_media.pdf

86. Sexton S, Natale R. Risks and benefits of pacifiers. Am Fam Physician 2009;79(8):681–5.

87.   CDC - Data and Statistics - Sleep and Sleep Disorders [Internet]. 2017 [cited 2018 Jun 26];Available from: https://www.cdc.gov/sleep/data_statistics.html

88.   Kostrzewa-Janicka J, Jurkowski P, Zycinska K, Przybyłowska D, Mierzwińska-Nastalska E. Sleep-Related Breathing Disorders and Bruxism. Adv Exp Med Biol 2015;873:9–14.

89.   Jokubauskas L, Baltrušaitytė A. Relationship between obstructive sleep apnoea syndrome and sleep bruxism: a systematic review. J Oral Rehabil 2017;44(2):144–53.

90.   Chervin RD, Dillon JE, Bassetti C, Ganoczy DA, Pituch KJ. Symptoms of sleep disorders, inattention, and hyperactivity in children. Sleep 1997;20(12):1185–92.

91.   Wu J, Gu M, Chen S, Chen W, Ni K, Xu H, et al. Factors related to pediatric obstructive sleep apnea-hypopnea syndrome in children with attention deficit hyperactivity disorder in different age groups. Medicine 2017;96(42):e8281.

92.   Philby MF, Macey PM, Ma RA, Kumar R, Gozal D, Kheirandish-Gozal L. Reduced Regional Grey Matter Volumes in Pediatric Obstructive Sleep Apnea. Sci Rep 2017;7:44566.

93.   Macey PM, Kheirandish-Gozal L, Prasad JP, Ma RA, Kumar R, Philby MF, et al. Altered Regional Brain Cortical Thickness in Pediatric Obstructive Sleep Apnea. Front Neurol 2018;9:4.

94.   McNamara JA Jr, Lione R, Franchi L, Angelieri F, Cevidanes LHS, Darendeliler MA, et al. The role of rapid maxillary expansion in the promotion of oral and general health. Prog Orthod 2015;16:33.

95.   Guilleminault C, Monteyrol P-J, Huynh NT, Pirelli P, Quo S, Li K. Adeno-tonsillectomy and rapid maxillary distraction in pre-pubertal children, a pilot study. Sleep Breath 2011;15(2):173–7.

96.   Lehmann KJ, Nelson R, MacLellan D, Anderson P, Romao RLP. The role of adenotonsillectomy in the treatment of primary nocturnal enuresis in children: A systematic review. J Pediatr Urol 2018;14(1):53.e1–53.e8.

97.   Oral health in America: a report of the Surgeon General. J Calif Dent Assoc 2000;28(9):685–95.

98.   Bishara SE. Management of diastemas in orthodontics. Am J Orthod 1972;61(1):55–63.

99.   Khoury MJ, Cordero JF, Mulinare J, Opitz JM. Selected Midline Defect Associations: A Population Study. Pediatrics 1989;84(2):266–72.

100. Hirsch S, Sanchez H, Albala C, de la Maza MP, Barrera G, Leiva L, et al. Colon cancer in Chile before and after the start of the flour fortification program with folic acid. Eur J Gastroenterol Hepatol 2009;21(4):436–9.

101. Troen AM, Mitchell B, Sorensen B, Wener MH, Johnston A, Wood B, et al. Unmetabolized folic acid in plasma is associated with reduced natural killer cell cytotoxicity among postmenopausal women. J Nutr 2006;136(1):189–94.

102. Mills JL. Fortification of Foods with Folic Acid — How Much is Enough? N Engl J Med 2000;342(19):1442–5.

103. Brandalize APC, Bandinelli E, dos Santos PA, Roisenberg I, Schüler-Faccini L. Evaluation of C677T and A1298C polymorphisms of the MTHFR gene as maternal risk factors for Down syndrome and congenital heart defects. Am J Med Genet A 2009;149A(10):2080–7.

104. Imbard A, Benoist J-F, Blom HJ. Neural tube defects, folic acid and methylation. Int J Environ Res Public Health 2013;10(9):4352–89.

105. CDC. Data and Statistics | Autism Spectrum Disorder (ASD) | NCBDDD | CDC [Internet]. Centers for Disease Control and Prevention 2018 [cited 2018 Jun 25];Available from: https://www.cdc.gov/ncbddd/autism/data.html

106. Rogers AP. Exercises for the development of the muscles of the face, with a view to increasing their functional activity. Dental Cosmos LX 1918;59(857):e76.

107. Bonuck K, Freeman K, Chervin RD, Xu L. Sleep-disordered breathing in a population-based cohort: behavioral outcomes at 4 and 7 years. Pediatrics 2012;129(4):e857–65.

108. Camacho M, Certal V, Abdullatif J, Zaghi S, Ruoff CM, Capasso R, et al. Myofunctional Therapy to Treat Obstructive Sleep Apnea: A Systematic Review and Meta-analysis. Sleep 2015;38(5):669–75.

109.   Mindell JA, Owens JA. A Clinical Guide to Pediatric Sleep: Diagnosis and Management of Sleep Problems. Lippincott Williams & Wilkins; 2015.

110.   Proffit WR, Fields HW Jr, Sarver DM. Contemporary Orthodontics. Elsevier Health Sciences; 2006.

111.   Chiropractic care for children: Controversies and issues. Paediatr Child Health 2002;7(2):85–104.

112.   Lee AC, Li DH, Kemper KJ. Chiropractic care for children. Arch Pediatr Adolesc Med 2000;154(4):401–7.

113.   Fry LM. Chiropractic and breastfeeding dysfunction: A literature review. Journal of Clinical Chiropractic Pediatrics 2014;14(2):1151–5.

114.   Page P. Cervicogenic headaches: an evidence-led approach to clinical management. Int J Sports Phys Ther 2011;6(3):254–66.

115.   Mawji A, Vollman AR, Hatfield J, McNeil DA, Sauvé R. The incidence of positional plagiocephaly: a cohort study. Pediatrics 2013;132(2):298–304.

116.   Pérez-Machado JL, Rodríguez-Fuentes G. [Relationship between the prone position and achieving head control at 3 months]. An Pediatr 2013;79(4):241–7.

117.   Senju A, Shimono M, Tsuji M, Suga R, Shibata E, Fujino Y, et al. Inability of infants to push up in the prone position and subsequent development. Pediatr Int [Internet] 2018;Available from: http://dx.doi.org/10.1111/ped.13632

118.   Mukai S, Mukai C, Asaoka K. Congenital ankyloglossia with deviation of the epiglottis and larynx: symptoms and respiratory function in adults. Ann Otol Rhinol Laryngol 1993;102(8 Pt 1):620–4.

Appendix

These are the forms we use for diagnosis, examination, postoperative instructions, and follow-up appointments to aid those treating these babies and children.

Infant Questionnaire

(Adapted from Dr. Larry Kotlow, DDS)

Patient's Name _____ Birth date _____ Today's Date _____

Medical problems: _____ Heart disease _____ Bleeding disorders _____ Other_____

_____Male _____Female   Birth Weight _____   Present Weight _____   Birth Hospital_____

_____Vaginal birth _____C-Section Birth   Any birth complications? _____

Are you presently breastfeeding ____Yes ____No If no, how long since you stopped breastfeeding _____

Medical History:

1. Infants are usually given vitamin K at birth. Did your child receive the vitamin K shot? ____yes ____no
2. Was your infant premature? ___ Yes ___ No If yes, how many weeks? _____
3. Does your infant have any heart disease ___ Yes ___ No
4. Has your infant had any surgery? ___ Yes ___ No
5. **Has your infant experienced any of the following? Please check / circle / elaborate as needed.**

___ Shallow latch at breast or bottle
___ Falls asleep while eating
___Slides or pops on and off the nipple
___ Colic symptoms / Cries a lot
___ Reflux symptoms
___ Clicking or smacking noises when eating
___ Spits up often? Amount / Frequency_____
___ Gagging, choking, coughing when eating
___ Gassy (toots a lot) / Fussy often
___ Poor weight gain
___ Hiccups often
___ Lip curls under when nursing or taking bottle

___Gumming or chewing your nipple when nursing
___Pacifier falls out easily, doesn't like, won't stay in
___ Milk dribbles out of mouth when nursing/bottle
___ Short sleeping requiring feedings every 1-2hrs
___Snoring, noisy breathing or mouth breathing
___Feels like a full time job just to feed baby
___ Nose congested often
___ Baby is frustrated at the breast or bottle
How long does baby take to eat? _____
How often does baby eat? _____

6. Is your infant taking any medications? ___ Reflux ____Thrush Name of medication: _____

7. Has your infant had a prior surgery to correct the tongue or lip tie? If yes, when, where, and by whom?
_____

7. **Do you have any of the following signs or symptoms? Please check / circle / elaborate as needed.**

___ Creased, flattened or blanched nipples
___ Lipstick shaped nipples
___ Blistered or cut nipples
___ Bleeding nipples
Pain on a scale of 1-10 when first latching _____
Pain (1-10) during nursing: _____

___ Poor or incomplete breast drainage
___ Infected nipples or breasts
___Plugged ducts / engorgement / mastitis
___Nipple thrush
___ Using a nipple shield
___Baby prefers one side over other ___ (R/L)

Pediatrician _____ Phone number: _____

Lactation Consultant _____Phone number:_____

Who referred you to us? _____

Doctor's Signature _____

ALABAMA
TONGUE-TIE
CENTER

Infant Exam Form
(Adapted from Dr. Marty Kaplan, DDS)

Alabama Tongue-Tie Center Infant Assessment

Patient name : _____   Date: _____

(To Be Completed by Doctor)

Lip-Tie :   1   2   3   4
Presentation: Thin / Thick   Fibrous /Fleshy   Corded / Triangular

Lip evaluation:
- Callus or blisters present on upper lip? Y / N   Blisters on all lips? Y / N
- Upper lip curls up and out (flanges)? Y / N
- Upper lip stretches and rolls to the tip of the nose? Y / N
- Gums blanch when raising lip? Y / N
- Muscle tone: tight / flexible

Buccal Ties: None   Speed bump in cheek R / L   Limiting movement R / L

Tongue evaluation:
Classification of Tongue-Tie: 1- submucosal   2- sl. visible   3-almost to tip   4- to the tip
Anterior Tongue-Tie
- *Frenum Width*: None - slight- <1mm - moderate 2-5mm - severe > 5mm
    1. Barrier to finger sweep: small speed bump / moderate bump / fence
    2. Blanches gum when tongue retracts Y / N
    3. Sore or blister on tip of tongue Y / N
- Shape of Tongue: Notched / forked / cupped / heart-shaped / folds down / square / blades / rounded / blunted

Posterior Tongue-Tie:
  Finger Sweep - speed bump, moderate bump, fence, tenting, Eiffel tower, cord
  Appearance
    1. None
    2. Short < 5mm. / Medium 5-10 mm. /long > 10 mm.
    3. Lingual fiber: Thin/ Thick
    4. Fiber Inserts: anterior 1/3, middle 1/3 , posterior 1/3
    5. Deep /Hidden (seen with retraction / *Submucosal*)
- Finger suction: None - weak - strong -// clamp or bite - disorganized
- Retains pacifier? Y / N
- Tongue cycle: continuous progressive wave - short burst with prolonged rest - humping push   - pistons in and out – tremors - disorganized
- Tongue : posterior elevation - anterior point - sides curl – blades - cups
- Palate: Flat - Normal - High Arched - Bubble Palate
- Cleft : soft tissue/ boney

303

Infant Frenectomy Post-Op Form
(Adapted from Dr. Greg Notestine, DDS)

POST-OP INSTRUCTIONS FOR INFANT TONGUE-TIE RELEASE

Your goal is to have the frenum heal and re-form as far back as possible. You should do the stretches with the baby laying down on a bed or couch facing away from you like during the exam. There is a video on our website at www.TongueTieAL.com. Please follow-up within 7-10 days. **Begin doing the stretches the DAY AFTER the procedure.** Gloves (preferred) or clean hands with nails trimmed should be used for stretches.

1. If the lip was revised also, first put your fingers all the way in the fold of the lip and pull the lip up and out as high as possible, so you can see the white diamond and cover the nostrils. It may bleed slightly the first day or two, this is not a concern.
2. With one or two fingers, lift the tongue up and back just above the white diamond to put tension on the wound and hold for 10 seconds. It may bleed slightly the first day or two, this is not a concern.
3. The main issue is to open the "diamond" all the way up on the lip and especially the tongue. If you notice it is becoming tight, then stretch a little more to open it back up.
4. Repeat this ideally 6 times a day (4 minimum) (change up the time during the day).
5. Repeat this for 3 weeks.
6. At other times, play in your child's mouth a few times a day with clean fingers to avoid causing an oral aversion. Tickle the lips, the gums, or allow your child to suck your finger.
7. Tummy-Time as much as possible. Visit www.TummyTimeMethod.com for helpful tips.
8. The released area will form a wet scab after the first day. It will appear white and soft. It may change color to yellow or even green. This is not infection, but is just a scab in the mouth. The white / yellow area will get smaller each day lengthwise, but HEALING IS STILL HAPPENING! So even though the white scab will heal you must continue stretching or the new frenum will not be as long as possible and the surgery may need to be repeated. If you have any concerns, please contact our office.

Follow up with a lactation consultant is critical if nursing. Bottle-feeding babies will benefit from visiting a feeding therapist. A bodyworker (chiropractor, CST, etc.) is also very helpful. You should expect one better feed a day (two better feeds the second day, etc.). Sometimes there's an immediate difference in feeding, and sometimes it takes a few days. Skin to skin, warm baths, and soothing music can be very beneficial to calm the baby.

For pain make sure to give CHILDREN'S TYLENOL (160mg / 5mL) starting WHEN YOU GET HOME and for the next 2-3 days every 4-6 hours. For babies who weigh 6-8lbs give 40mg or 1.25mL, 9-11lb give 2mL. Babies 12-14lb can have 80mg or 2.5mL, 15-17lb give 3mL. If your child is 6mo old and 12-17lbs, you can give Infant's Motrin (ibuprofen) at 1.25mL (50mg). If your baby is refusing to nurse or seems to be in pain, please make sure the Tylenol dose is correct.

Your child's lip will swell up slightly that evening or the next day. It is normal and will go down after a day or two. The area will be sore for a few days, at one week look much better, and at two weeks look much better and almost normal.

If you have any questions, please call us at 205-419-4333, or Dr. Baxter's cell at ########.

Child Tongue-Tie Questionnaire

Patient's Name _____ Birthday _____ Age ____ Today's Date _____

Medical issues: _____ Medications taking: _____

Allergies: _____ Previous clip or release of tongue? _____ (date)

1. Has your child experienced any of the following issues? Please check or elaborate as needed.

Speech
__ Frustration with communication
__ Difficult to understand by parents
__ Difficult to understand by outsiders
__ % Percent of time you understand your child
__ Difficulty speaking fast
__ Difficulty getting words out (groping for words)
__ Trouble with sounds (which?)_____
__ Speech delay (when?)_____
__ Stuttering
__ Speech harder to understand in long sentences
__ Speech therapy (how long)_____
__ Mumbling or speaking softly
__ "Baby Talk"

Nursing or Bottle-Feeding Issues as a Baby
__ Painful nursing or shallow latch
__ Poor weight gain
__ Reflux or spitting up
__ Unable to hold pacifier
__ Milk dribbling out of mouth
__ Poor Supply
__ Nipple shield required for nursing
__ Clicking or smacking noise when eating
__ Other:

Other related issues
__ Neck or shoulder pain or tension
__ TMJ Pain, clicking, or popping
__ Headaches or migraines
__ Strong gag reflex
__ Mouth open /mouth breathing during the day
__ Tonsils or adenoids removed previously
__ Ear tubes previously
__ Reflux (medicated or not)
__ ADHD / ADD
__ Constipation

Feeding
__ Frustration when eating
__ Difficulty transitioning to solid foods
__ Slow eater (doesn't finish meals)
__ Grazes on food throughout the day
__ Packing food in cheeks like a chipmunk
__ Picky with textures (which?)_____
__ Choking or gagging on food
__ Spits out food
__ Other:

Sleep issues
__ Sleeps in strange positions
__ Kicks and flails around at night
__ Wakes easily or often
__ Wets the bed
__ Wakes up tired and not refreshed
__ Grinds teeth while sleeping
__ Sleeps with mouth open
__ Snores while sleeping (how often) _____
__ Gasps for air or stops breathing (sleep apnea)

Anything else we need to know:

Pediatrician _____

Speech Therapist _____

Who referred you to us? _____

Doctor's Signature _____

ALABAMA TONGUE-TIE CENTER

Child Post-Operative Instructions

(Adapted from Dr. Greg Notestine, DDS)

POST-OP INSTRUCTIONS FOR FRENECTOMY

Lingual Frenectomy (tongue-tie):

Your goal is to have the frenum heal and re-form as far back as possible.

1. With a clean or gloved finger, lift the tongue at the top of the diamond in the middle of the tongue. Your goal is to see the whole diamond open up and lengthen. It may bleed slightly when it is stretched or re-opened. This is not a concern. Begin doing this the morning after treatment. Try to make a game of it if possible and keep it playful.
2. Repeat this 3 times a day, at various times during the day for 3 weeks.
3. Encourage the child to move the tongue as much as possible by sticking it out and holding for 10 sec, out to the left, right, open wide and lift up, make clicking noises, and clean off the teeth. Do these exercises as often as possible, but try for 4 times a day.
4. The released area will form a wet scab after the first day. It will appear white or yellow and soft because it is wet. This area is what you will be pressing against. The healing will be happening under the scab, just like a scrape anywhere else on your body. The white area will get smaller each day, but healing is still happening! So even though the white scab will heal you MUST continue the stretching or the new frenum will not be as long as possible and the surgery may need to be repeated.

Labial Frenum (lip-tie):

The goal is for the frenum to heal and re-form as high as possible.

1. Pull the lip up as high as possible, high enough to press against the nose. You want to see the whole white diamond open up. Press gently but firmly against the wound to massage it and keep the diamond open. It may bleed slightly when this is done, but this is not a concern. Try to make a game of it if possible and keep it playful.
2. Repeat 3 times a day, at various times during the day for 3 weeks.
3. The released area will form a wet scab after the first day. It will appear white or yellow and soft because it is wet. This area is what you will be pressing against. The healing will be happening under the scab, just like a scrape anywhere else on your body. The white area will get smaller each day, but healing is still happening! So even though the white scab will heal you MUST continue the stretching or the new frenum will not be as long as possible and the surgery may need to be repeated.

The child can eat whatever foods he or she can tolerate. Pain relief is needed the first few days. Give Motrin (Ibuprofen) or Tylenol as directed on the package based on weight. If the lip-tie was released, the child's lip may swell up slightly that evening or the next day. It is normal and will go down after a day or two. The wound will be sore for a few days, at one week look much better, and at two weeks look almost normal. A slight fever is normal the first day. They should eat and sleep normally. If you're concerned it is growing back together, come back for a visit or email a picture. Follow-up with a myofunctional therapist and bodyworker (Chiropractor, CST) is recommended for full rehabilitation.

If you have any questions, please call us at 205-419-4333, or Dr. Baxter's cell at #########.

Child Follow-Up Questionnaire

Patient's Name _____ Date of Birth: _____

Today's Date _____ Days Since Procedure : _____

ALABAMA
TONGUE-TIE
CENTER

Has your child experienced improvement or changes in any of the following issues?

INSTRUCTIONS: Please mark any previous issues that saw improvement.

Speech
___ Easier to communicate
___ Easier to understand by parents
___ Easier to understand by outsiders
___ Understand more words your child says.
___ Easier to speak fast
___ Easier to get words out (not groping for words)
___ Easier with sounds (which?)_____
___ New words? _____
___ Less Stuttering
___ Speech easier to understand in long sentences
___ Less mumbling or speaking softly
___ Less "Baby Talk"

Feeding
___ Less frustration when eating
___ Easier to eat solid foods
___ Eating faster
___ Finishing meals better
___ Less grazing on food throughout the day
___ Less packing food in cheeks like a chipmunk
___ Less picky with textures (which?)_____
___ Less choking or gagging on food
___ Less spiting out food
___ Other:

Sleep issues
___ Less sleeping in strange positions
___ Less kicking and moving around at night
___ Sleeping deeper and waking less
___ Less wetting the bed
___ Wakes up less tired and more refreshed
___ Less grinding teeth while sleeping
___ Less sleeping with mouth open
___ Less snoring while sleeping
___ Less gasping for air or stopping breathing

Other related issues
___ Less neck or shoulder pain or tension
___ Less TMJ Pain, clicking, or popping
___ Less headaches or migraines
___ Less strong gag reflex
___ Less mouth open/mouth breathing during the day
___ Less reflux
___ Better attention span
___ Less hyperactivity issues
___ Less constipation

How much improvement did you see from the release? (circle one):

Speech

Significant improvement / Moderate improvement / Slight Improvement / No Change   N/A

Feeding

Significant improvement / Moderate improvement / Slight Improvement / No Change   N/A

Sleep

Significant improvement / Moderate improvement / Slight Improvement / No Change   N/A

307

About the Authors

Richard Baxter, DMD, MS

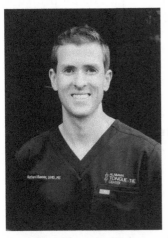 Dr. Richard Baxter is a board-certified pediatric dentist and Diplomate of the American Board of Laser Surgery. He lives in Birmingham, AL, with his wife Tara, and three daughters Hannah, Noelle, and Molly. He is the founder and owner of Shelby Pediatric Dentistry and the Alabama Tongue-Tie Center, where he uses the CO_2 laser to release oral restrictions that are causing nursing, speech, dental, sleep and feeding issues. He had a tongue-tie himself, and all three of his girls were treated for tongue and lip-tie at birth, so for him, this field is a personal one. In his free time, he enjoys spending time with his family, reading, and outdoor activities. Dr. Baxter also participates in many overseas dental mission trips and is currently working on several projects related to tongue-ties involving research and education.

Megan Musso, MA, CCC-SLP

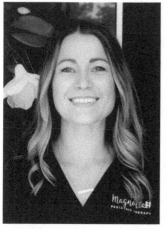

Megan Musso is a certified and licensed Speech-Language Pathologist and the founder and owner of Magnolia Pediatric Therapy in Lake Charles, Louisiana. She graduated with her bachelor's and master's degrees from Louisiana State University and has since pursued her passion for pediatric feeding and early intervention. Megan's experiences working with the pediatric population include treating feeding disorders in infants and children with tethered oral tissues, medically fragile infants, adolescents with special needs, and normally developing children with oral aversion or "picky eating." In her spare time, Megan enjoys a good cup of coffee, traveling with her husband, and coaching track and field at Barbe High School.

Lauren Hughes, MS, CCC-SLP

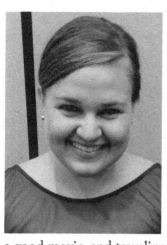

Lauren Hughes is a certified Speech-Language Pathologist and owner of Expressions Pediatric Therapy in Birmingham, AL. She received her master's degree from the University of Southern Mississippi and has pursued training to further her understanding of feeding, oral motor, speech, and language disorders to provide the best quality services for her clients. In her free time, Lauren enjoys reading, spending time with friends, watching a good movie, and traveling to new places.

Lisa Lahey, RN, IBCLC

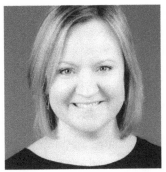

Lisa has worked in maternal child health as a registered nurse and lactation consultant for 22 years, first in the hospital setting of Labor and Delivery, postpartum, NICU and newborn nursery. An IBCLC for 19 years, Lisa has a special interest in tethered oral tissues and myofunctional therapy, and has taken many trainings and courses beyond her baccalaureate nursing degree to provide expertise to her patients. Lisa now provides lactation consults and holistic modalities for complex breastfeeding issues in her private practice, Advanced Breastfeeding Care. Lisa also works in a functional orthodontic office in Indianapolis, IN, providing myofunctional assessment and therapy to babies, children, and adults. Lisa teaches an IBCLC Master Class course with other colleagues on tie assessment and oral rehabilitation. She enjoys traveling with her husband and her 5 children to National Parks to unplug and enjoy nature.

Paula Fabbie, RDH, BS, COM

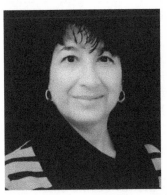

Paula Fabbie, RDH, BS, COM (board-certified orofacial myologist) consults, lectures, and writes articles on orofacial myofunctional disorders (OMDs) and how they impact overall health and sleep. Paula offers a unique perspective on time-proven oral rest posture principles combined with evidenced-based science to assist her patients in achieving myofunctional goals and functional breathing. She operates Paula Fabbie, LLC, where she provides myofunctional services.

Marty Lovvorn, DC

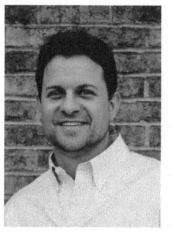

Dr. Marty Lovvorn is the founder and lead Gonstead doctor of Precision Chiropractic of Alabama. Dr. Lovvorn is a graduate of Auburn University (B.S.) and Life University (D.C). He is dedicated to specializing in the world-renowned Gonstead Technique and focuses on pediatric development, pregnancy and prenatal care, athletic injury recovery, and adult health. He is passionate about making a lasting impact through the education and application of principled chiropractic care. Dr. Lovvorn, his wife, and two children live in Birmingham, AL, where they enjoy outdoor recreational activities and family time.

Michelle Emanuel, OTR/L, NBCR, CST, CIMI, RYT200

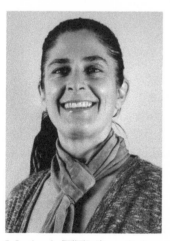

Michelle is a neonatal/pediatric occupational therapist, national board certified reflexologist, certified craniosacral therapist, certified infant massage instructor, and a registered yoga teacher specializing in the precrawling infant. For 17 years, she worked at Cincinnati Children's Hospital Medical Center, in both inpatient/NICU and outpatient/development realms. During this time, Michelle developed the TummyTime!™ Method (TTM) to help parents and babies overcome challenges and love tummy time. She also educates, certifies, and mentors professionals to become certified in TTM. For the past few years,

Michelle has been in full-time private practice, evaluating and treating babies with cranial nerve dysfunction (CND), tethered oral tissues (TOTs) and precrawling baby oral motor/developmental concerns. She also travels extensively teaching her curriculum, collaborates and co-teaches with other TOTs professionals, and is on the teaching staff of the Academy of Orofacial Myofunctional Therapy. Michelle lives in Cincinnati with her three children, a son in college and two daughters, both in high school.

Tongue-Tied Academy

An Online Course That Helps You Identify & Treat Oral Restrictions With Confidence.

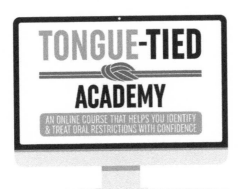

In this comprehensive online course, Dr. Richard Baxter explains in detail how to evaluate, diagnose, and treat patients with oral restrictions. A thorough background of tongue-ties and the effects on patients throughout the lifespan is discussed, as well as dozens of cases explained and the latest research summarized. A business perspective module details how to train team members, billing and insurance issues, and how to get started treating tongue-tie patients. Finally, full patient treatment videos of our consultation, treatment, and follow-up methods help providers virtually observe our office without having to travel or close their offices. Sign up today to start learning on your own time and begin treating patients with confidence.

Learn More and Get Started at www.TongueTiedAcademy.com

Made in USA - Kendallville, IN
95867_9781732508200
09.19.2023 1349